THE PSORIASIS HANDBOOK
A Self-Help Guide

by

Muriel K. MacFarlane, RN, MA

United Research Publishers

Published by United Research Publishers

ISBN 1-887053-01-8

Library of Congress Catalog Card Number 95-61640

Printed and bound in the United States of America

The information in this book is not intended to replace the advice of your physician. You should consult your doctor regarding any medical condition which concerns you. The material presented in this book is intended to inform and educate the reader with a view to making some intelligent choices in pursuing the goal of living your life in a healthy, vigorous manner. Neither the author nor the publisher assumes any responsibility or liability for the judgements or decisions any reader might make as a result of reading this publication.

Book design by The Final Draft, Encinitas, CA

Cover design by The Art Department, Encinitas, CA

Order additional copies from:
United Research Publishers
P.O. Box 2344
Leucadia, CA 92024

Full 30-day money back guarantee if not satisfied.

CONTENTS

Introduction

Despite the feeling that a lot of people have, of wanting to avoid someone with scaly and flaking skin, the truth is that you probably know someone with psoriasis. Psoriasis is one of the most common skin disorders--it affects one in every 50 adults. What the dictionary definition doesn't describe is the emotional and psychological effect of having this visible and disturbing ailment. Sufferers feel embarrassed and unattractive.

As one young man pointed out, "People ask you, 'What is that?' in a way that implies you should be cleaner or do something to get your skin fixed. Upon being introduced to me, after shaking my hand and looking at my forehead, I've actually had people wipe their hand off and back away with a disgusted expression on their face."

In his book *At War with My Skin*, writer John Updike reflected on his lifelong battle with psoriasis. His suffering from the fluctuating and seemingly shameful condition caused him to cultivate habits of concealment and endless self-examination. He writes that "psoriasis has the volatility of a disease, the sense of another presence co-occupying your body, and singling you out from the happy herds of healthy, normal mankind. . . ." He knew that he could suffer an outbreak at any time--often inconvenient times--and it took Updike a lifetime to come to the conclusion that having the disease encouraged courage and independence in choices about career, marriage, family, and travel. Many others are not as brave or insightful as Updike, however, and spend a lifetime in self-blame and self-disgust, disabled and depressed. To have a very visible affliction is to find oneself the victim of stigma and discrimination. To have psoriasis is to suffer the frustration of treatments that don't work. To experience physicians who are less than sympathetic because they consider it nothing more than an inconvenience that isn't life-threatening. To talk with physicians who become discouraged with a patient who has a disease that seems to be incurable and therefore is disappointing to the doctor. To find that there are remissions and then recurrences, and not understand why or how this happens. To hear about folk remedies that have worked miracles for others and then find they are useless when you try them. To have almost no one to talk to about the condition, and be rebuffed by employers, friends and family. To wake up daily to a routine of self-examination, looking for any sign of the condition's disappearance. To suffer the unbearable itching and the disapproval of others when the scaling and flakes appear. To experience interactions with others who believe you should be able to do something about your appearance. To constantly feel unattractive and undesirable, lacking in self-worth, diminished in self-esteem because of a skin condition that appears to have no cure, is to become disabled and depressed. This could be a definition of psoriasis.

But it doesn't have to be. This book is for all those individuals who feel overwhelmed by their disease and its symptoms. Hopefully it will provide some understandable information about the disease--what it is, what can be done to treat it, and how you can live your life more fully while coping with the skin condition known as psoriasis. Treatments are changing. Researchers are currently developing newer treatments and improving on older ones that have been found to have some validity. Genetic factors are being explored.

Knowledge is your best defense against any attacker. Knowledge of how psoriasis develops and what you can do to limit its progress, effective ways of coping to minimize its discomforts and distresses, are the tools this book is designed to provide. With understandable information about medical treatments, psychological counseling, support groups, stress reduction, and home therapy, you can limit the effect psoriasis has on your life.

1

Jennifer's story

Jennifer was a popular high school teenager. A cheerleader, a class officer, member of a number of clubs, a homecoming princess; she was active and busy. She had already worked part-time as a model, and she thought she might want to be a cheerleader for one of the major football or basketball teams, like the Laker Girls, when she graduated. She took a variety of dance classes with that thought in the back of her mind. The 5-foot-5, 120 pound beauty was probably the most popular girl in school. The boys fell all over themselves whenever she flashed her drop-dead smile. Jennifer's mother knew nothing of this Laker Girl dream of Jennifer's, and she always talked about her ambitions for Jennifer to go to college and maybe to law school one day.

"Sure, Mom, that sounds great," Jennifer would say, but she always thought that she would be a professional cheerleader first, maybe only for a couple of years, before she got serious about hitting the books at college. A lot of her friends were going directly to college, but Jennifer had other plans.

During the summer vacation between her junior and senior years, she came home from a dance class with a sore throat and a headache. After a week or two of feeling awful, she was diagnosed first with strep throat and then with infectious mononucleosis. Her friends kidded her a lot about catching the "kissing disease," but a couple of weeks later, after resting in bed and taking aspirin for the headaches, Jennifer was feeling a lot better. By the time school began in the fall, she had almost forgotten that she had been sick at all that summer.

Always conscious of her appearance, Jennifer was disturbed to find a lot of silvery flakes on her shoulders. "Dandruff. Ugh!" She ran right out and got herself some dandruff shampoo and began to wash her hair vigorously every day.

"Mom, this shampoo isn't doing anything for this dandruff, it seems to be getting worse instead of better," she complained.

"Let me take a look at your scalp," her mother said.

Jennifer turned obediently and bent her head down. Her mother parted the long blond hair at several spots and then lifted her hair from the back of her neck. "Good heavens, you must have gotten scabies or something. I can't believe the way your scalp looks behind your ears!," said her mother.

"Oh, Mom, where would I get scabies?" laughed Jennifer. "You are exaggerating, as usual."

When the rash began to appear at the front of her scalp and the flakes were falling into her eyebrows, Jennifer cut bangs to cover her forehead. She continued to shampoo her hair regularly and tried all the different shampoos she found in the drugstore--but nothing seemed to make much difference. She continued to throw herself into her dance and cheerleading practice sessions but secretly she worried--and avoided wearing dark colors that would show the flakes on her clothes or hair styles that revealed too much of her hairline.

At practice after school one afternoon, the girls all sat down on the gym bleachers to have a drink.

"What's that on your elbow?" said one of the other cheerleaders.

"Where?" asked Jennifer. She pulled her arm around so she could look at it and was dismayed to see the already all-too-familiar flaking skin on her elbow. That evening, she showed the spot to her mother and they both realized she had something more than dandruff, more than just a temporary rash. After a sleepless night, they made an appointment to see the doctor.

It was not long after examining her scalp and her elbows that Jennifer's doctor gave her a diagnosis. "It's psoriasis, a chronic and recurrent dermatological disease."

Jennifer had never heard of the condition before, but her mother had. "Oh, no, Jennifer keeps herself very clean. She couldn't possibly have any kind of a skin disease," exclaimed her mother.

Over the next five years Jennifer would learn a lot about this skin condition. And. . . while she was learning just what psoriasis was, she was learning just what having it would mean to her life. She would also learn how it affected a lot of other people who were just as ignorant as she had been about the skin condition and what having it meant.

History of psoriasis

Psoriasis originates from the Greek word *psora* which means to itch. There have been times when psoriasis has been known as the baker's itch, the grocer's itch and the bricklayer's itch--obviously a lot of people in the past have had it. Galen, the Greek physician and medical writer of the second century AD, is thought to have named the condition. In early medicine, psoriasis was also confused with leprosy, a word with its origin in the word to scale, referring to the silvery flakes of skin. Victims of psoriasis were often sent to leper colonies, cast out from their homes or even burned at the stake as heretics or witches.

This lack of knowledge persisted for hundreds

of years until the nineteenth century when another famous scientist, Ferdinand von Hebra, an Austrian dermatologist and founder of the histological school of dermatology, realized that psoriasis was a separate condition. Although Hebra gave a differential diagnosis, it didn't make much of a change in the way individuals with the condition were treated. The medical community was unable to offer much in the way of treatment, and non-sufferers continued to treat sufferers as if they were lepers--with avoidance and ridicule.

One of the earliest recorded treatments was described by Thomas Bateman in 1819. He suggested the use of mercury, a purgative, some cream, a topical application of oil of almonds and a mild anti-inflammatory.

Radcliff Crocker in 1893 used arsenic given orally as a treatment, and found that it took up to three months to work, hopefully without poisoning his clients.

The treatment of psoriasis has come a long way since the nineteenth century, and with the current interest in genetic engineering it does seem hopeful that better treatments and possibly a cure might be on the horizon.

Psoriasis defined

Dorland's *Illustrated Medical Dictionary* defines psoriasis as "skin disease of many varieties, characterized by the formation of scaly red patches on the extensor surfaces of the body." The dictionary goes on with further definitions: *p. annularis*, psoriasis in ring-shaped patches; *p. arthropathica*, a form associated with chronic arthritis; *p. buccalis*, leukoplakia buccalis, in which the lesions are formed upon the mucous membrane of the cheeks; *p. circinata*, another form of annularis; *p. diffusa*, a form in which there is more or less coalescence of large contiguous (touching upon each other) lesions; *p. discoides*, occurring in solid, persistent patches; *p. figurata*, with lesions in curved, linear patterns; *p. follicularis*, a form in which small scaly lesions are located at the openings of sebaceous and sweat glands; *p. guttata*, a form occurring in small, distinct, and irregular patches; *p. gyrata*, a form with patches having a serpentine arrangement; *p. inverterata*, a form with confluent (flowing together) lesions and with thickening and hardening of the skin; *p. linguae*, (the tongue) leukoplakia buccalis; *p. nummularis*, a form in circular patches which resemble small coins; *p. osteacea*, a form in thick tough patches covered with scales resembling the outside of an oyster shell; *p. palmaris et plantaris*, a syphiloderm of the palms or soles;

p. punctata, a variety in which the lesions consist of minute, red, pinhead-shaped papules, often surmounted with pearly scales; *pustular p.*, a form in which the lesions are covered with small pustules; *p. rupioides*, a form in which rupia-like crusts (vesicles) are formed, which then become scabby); *p. universalis*, a form with lesions over the entire body. A lot of definitions--obviously psoriasis comes in a lot of differing forms.

2

The types of psoriasis

There are five main forms of psoriasis:

Common plaque psoriasis

This most common type of psoriasis is also known as *psoriasis vulgaris* or *nummular* (coin-like) and is the type that 80 to 90 percent of all individuals who have psoriasis experience. It appears as raised red, or even darker, round or oval scaling patches. On the lower legs the plaques can appear almost purple in color. The two descriptive adjectives--chronic and plaque--refer to the fact that it tends to persist for a long time and occurs in patches which may vary in size, from those as small as a dot to patches as large as a dinner plate. As they enlarge, they may merge into one another, sometimes covering large areas of the body. The scales, which are silvery and thick, occur most frequently on the elbows, knees, scalp and lower back, but all parts of the skin may occasionally be subject to plaques. When the scales are scratched off, small bleeding points remain. These bleeding points are the enlarged blood vessels in the dermis.

One indicator of the fact that this is a condition of the body rather than an insult from the outside, such as a blow, is that psoriasis almost always appears in a symmetrical form--that is, if it is on one elbow it will also appear on the other. This demonstrates the fact that this is a general disorder of the skin cells and not something affecting that area of the body from the outside, such as an infection in a cut or an allergic dermitis.

Itching is one of the most disturbing symptoms of psoriasis, causing much discomfort to the sufferer and prompting others to notice the condition. The itching is related to the degree of inflammation or redness of the skin that surrounds the plaques. Itching appears to be lessened with treatment: as inflammation is reduced, itching is reduced.

Psoriasis can appear for the first time anywhere, but it seems to start first on the elbows and knees. Almost two-thirds find these are the beginning sites, and for half of those these will be the only sites of the condition. It is not known why this occurs but it is thought that friction over a bony prominence is the initiating factor. Following these two sites, the scalp is the most frequent. Three-fourths of individuals with psoriasis have it on the scalp, elbows and knees.

The scalp is one of the most difficult areas to

disguise as the white silvery flakes appear on the shoulders and collars, and it is one of the most difficult areas to treat. Hair makes the application of ointments difficult and it also protects the scalp from sunlight, which is known to lessen the condition.

Other common sites are the lower back, around the ears and in the umbilicus. It is very unusual to have psoriasis in other locations without it first beginning in the areas of the elbows, knees or scalp.

The progression of the condition and its symptoms vary from individual to individual. Itching, while common, does not affect everyone. Scaling varies from person to person also. Seasonal differences appear to be related to the amount of natural sunlight available, with winter being the worst season and summer the best.

Guttate psoriasis

This type of psoriasis is the type which frequently starts in childhood or in the teens and is much less common than chronic plaque psoriasis. It often occurs after a brief illness with a sore throat from streptococcal type infection. *Streptococcus* is a germ that is everywhere, on our skin and throughout our environment. When it does cause an infection, it is usually stopped by our tonsils, our first line of defense in the lymph system. Treatment of a strep throat or other strep infection with penicillin is quite effective. Where there is a genetic history of psoriasis it is best to treat such strep infections early, particularly in children. However, such psoriasis occurs only in those who have inherited the tendency to develop the condition, and it usually follows two to four weeks after exposure. There will be a sudden occurrence of many tiny patches scattered all over the body, like tiny raindrops (guttate means drop-shaped) which usually is not accompanied by scales, except in the scalp. The patches are much smaller than those of plaque psoriasis and tend to be scattered all over, with the main affected areas usually being the trunk and tops of the limbs. Only 10 percent of psoriasis seems to be of this type and it occurs most frequently in children and young adults.

This type of psoriasis will frequently resolve on its own, but occasionally it is stubborn and can become common psoriasis.

Guttate psoriasis can be quite severe, and although it may cover large parts of the body, it responds very rapidly when exposed to ultraviolet light and other forms of treatment. Sometimes this will be the only outbreak the individual may have. However, localized patches or plaques may develop later in the individual's life.

Pustular psoriasis

Localized pustular psoriasis

One of the more unusual forms of psoriasis, it is often found on the palms of the hands or the soles of the feet. It looks quite different than some of the other forms, and will consist of multiple small pustules: brown or white small dots which are surrounded by reddened and inflamed skin. This pus does not represent an infection of any kind, but indicates that the skin is inflamed. It can be very uncomfortable when walking or working with the hands. In addition, it is possible to have the plaques and patches of regular psoriasis at the same time.

When the hands and feet alone are the areas affected, it is found only on the palms of the hands and soles of the feet. In this type, the pustules develop as flat, yellow, pus-appearing spots which eventually dry up, turn brown and then peel off. The skin is often very dry and has a tendency to crack, which is very painful. The condition is slow to respond to treatment.

Generalized pustular psoriasis

This very severe form of psoriasis can be caused by a number of things, including infections and certain medications (such as lithium or system cortisones). It can occur as a reaction to a severe sunburn. The individual will feel sick and may have a fever. When this type of psoriasis begins, the areas often become bright red, painful and appear swollen. The start of the condition is often on the legs, and any moisturizer or emollient can make the condition more uncomfortable.

The usual treatment for this type is oral etretinate. Although this form of psoriasis is quite rare, it can require hospitalization.

Erythrodermic psoriasis

This type of psoriasis completely covers the entire body, and is also known as exfoliative psoriasis or generalized psoriasis. Almost the entire area of the skin can be involved, becoming red, itchy and swollen. Sometimes there are raw areas which ooze fluid. Other parts of the body may be involved, including the eyes, the lining of the mouth and inside the nose. Erythrodermic psoriasis may begin as common psoriasis and become gradually more extensive, or appear quite suddenly as a flare of red inflamed skin because of a reaction to treatment. Quite often there is no reason that is apparent. Because such large areas of skin are involved, the individual may feel extremely uncomfortable since there may be difficulties in controlling body temperature because of heat and fluid losses, quite similar to the way the skin behaves after severe burns. The individual can feel extremely weak and cold. Because the surface of the body is open, the individual is vulnerable to infections. Older individuals or people with heart or kidney disease may experience an increase in heart rate due to the increased blood supply flowing to the severely inflamed skin. Fortunately, fewer than 10 percent of individuals have this type of the disease.

This type of psoriasis is difficult to treat. In many cases it is difficult to take a skin biopsy and difficult to diagnose. The general health of the patient requires attention with warmth, fluids and skin care.

Flexural and genital psoriasis

This type of psoriasis can occur in conjunction with some of the more common types of the disease and can create great discomfort when skin folds cause areas of the body to rub against one another. When the condition occurs in the genital area it can be a cause of extreme discomfort. It may be troubling to sexual partners who perhaps do not know what the skin condition is and may be worried that it is a sexually transmitted disease and/or that it may be contagious.

Overweight individuals more frequently are troubled with skin fold irritations because their skin tends to fold over itself more frequently.

3

The cause of psoriasis

The cause of psoriasis is not yet fully understood but many researchers are working on discovering why it occurs and just who is prone to the skin condition, and searching for potential cures.

In psoriasis, new cells rush to form more skin in three days instead of the normal 28 to 30 days. This abnormal cell growth causes the excessive skin cells to pile up with nowhere to go except to the surface, where they form red, scaly plaques or lesions that are covered with a silvery-white scale composed of dead skin cells. The main characteristics of psoriasis are intense itching and painful, dry and cracking skin. Although the disorder is chronic, it can be controlled or made to go into remission. Mark A. Everett, head of the department of dermatology at the University of Oklahoma Health Sciences Center, notes that psoriasis occurs in all segments of the population, including at least five million Americans.

Science has examined the behavior of both the dermis and the epidermis as the culprit in psoriasis. In the condition there are changes in both layers, the epidermis (outer) and the dermis (inner) layer. It appears that the initial change then initiates the next step, in a domino-type reaction until the patch of plaque known as psoriasis appears.

If the cause takes place in the epidermis, there is uncontrolled growth of the outer skin cells. Support for this theory comes from research which shows that the epidermal cells divide and grow much more rapidly than normal epidermal cells (dividing at least twenty-five times as rapidly). Cells move from the deepest layer of the epidermis in only four days, requiring more nutrition, so surrounding blood vessels grow more rapidly and larger to provide that nutrition. As this occurs, white blood cells come in to try to control the skin growth.

If the cause takes place in the dermis, which is below the epidermis, it is thought that the changes in the upper skin cells take place because of repair and growth instructions which come from the blood cells in the dermis.

There is a highly specialized cell found in the epidermis and occasionally in the dermis. It is part of the immune system, acting as a guard against foreign substances. It locates foreign substances and points them out to the immune system which then initiates a reaction to eliminate or destroy the foreign substance. In psoriasis these cells are present in the skin in larger numbers than in so-called normal skin and are more active. They are surrounded by special white blood cells which are part of the immune system and they release chemicals which act as messengers telling other cells what they should do. If they spot a foreign substance, such as a germ, they find it and proceed to eliminate it from the body by increased activity which, in turn, produces the greater activity of the epidermis.

Both of these theories have researchers examining ways to control cell behavior in both the epidermis and the dermis.

Other research is examining the chemicals produced by the white blood cells and the epidermal and dermal cells as the messengers which initiate the changes in the skin.

A gene involved in the susceptibility to psoriasis was recently found in the distal region of a human chromosome. In a study by James Tomfohrde, Alan Silverman and Robert Barnes reported in *Science*, the researchers demonstrated that psoriasis susceptibility is due to variation at a single major genetic locus. This is very good news for genetic researchers as well as sufferers because this means that, with further investigation into genetic engineering, it may be possible to alter this genetic predisposition which could result in the elimination of the skin disorder entirely.

Researchers have long suspected that an autoimmune malfunction might be at the root of the disease, but have never been able to prove that concept. Using the prior developments pioneered by Dr. John Murphy at University Hospital in Boston, a team under Dr. James Kreuger, a researcher and assistant professor in the Laboratory for Investigative Dermatology at Rockefeller University in New York, took a molecule that causes diphtheria and modified it genetically. They then introduced this genetically engineered molecule into volunteers where it appeared to alter the immune response. Further studies are now underway to determine the long-term success of such a treatment.

Is psoriasis a serious condition?

The severity of psoriasis is measured by the extent of body surface affected and the location on the body. If 10 percent of the body surface is involved, physicians consider it a mild case. Ten to 30 percent is considered moderate; and more than 30 percent, severe. The palm of the hand equals one percent when measuring body surface. Severity can be measured additionally in terms of its emotional impact on the individual.

Psoriasis can involve a small area of the body and have a serious impact on the individual's ability to function properly. When it is confined to the palms of the hands and the soles of the feet you might consider this a very small area of the body, but when located here it can be severe enough to be physically disabling. The Social Security Administration grants disability to approximately 400 individuals annually who find their condition sufficiently limiting to prevent them from working or performing the requirements of day to day self-care.

For the majority, it remains limited to one or a few patches on the skin and the most common areas for it to appear are on the scalp, elbows, knees and trunk of the body, although it can appear anywhere.

When the disease affects major body surfaces, a variety of physical problems can occur such as intense itching, pain, dry and cracked skin and swelling. These types of physical problems can affect both movement and flexibility.

In a few cases, severe types of psoriasis, such as pustular or erythrodermic, can elevate body temperature to the point of placing strain on some of the internal organs of the body such as the heart and the kidneys. In these instances, hospitalization is required to avoid complications which may threaten the person's life. Approximately 400 people die yearly of some of the complications of psoriasis-related illnesses.

The emotional impact can be as serious as the physical impact. Because others consider the scales and flaky skin unsightly, their reaction to the condition can contribute to low self-confidence and self-esteem. The result may be feelings of embarrassment, anger, depression and guilt.

The effects of injury

It has been observed that psoriasis will occur at the site of an injury to the skin, whether that be a small scratch or the scar line following surgery. Individuals who are undergoing radiation treatment for cancer, a severe sunburn, or any other injury which interrupts the integrity of the skin's surface may find that the site has become an opportunity for psoriasis to arise. This phenomenon is known as the Koebner phenomenon and is well known among physicians who treat the skin condition. This would indicate that the body's reaction to injury and automatic response to insult to the skin's epidermal system is to develop a psoriatic lesion.

What is a psoriasis remission?

Psoriasis goes through cycles of improvements and then flare-ups. It can go into spontaneous remission for reasons that are not yet understood, although stress has been implicated in flares and periods of quietude in the patient's life have been noted to be related to remissions.

One study showed that two out of five individuals with psoriasis have stated that they have experienced remissions, lasting from one to as long as 64 years.

4

The skin is an organ

We look at someone and say, "Doesn't she have nice skin." Usually when such a comment is made we are only looking at the person's face. Many people see the skin as nothing more than a simple thin covering that either has blemishes or wrinkles or those age spots that nobody likes--but the skin is definitely more than that. It is more than a sack that keeps the body together, holding the bones and internal organs in place, and protecting them from harm. A detailed observation of the skin reveals that it is quite complex in structure and performs a number of vital functions. The skin is essential for survival, but in addition, the skin is the body's "mood ring," revealing the emotions. We blush when we are embarrassed. We go pale when we are frightened. Anger or exertion makes our faces bright red--and stress is often written all over our face.

Any grouping of tissues that perform a specific function is known as an organ. The skin is an organ, just like the kidneys, the heart or the lungs, because it consists of tissues that are structurally joined together to perform specific activities. A detailed observation of the skin reveals that it is quite complex in structure but more essentially, it is vital for survival in a number of ways.

The skin is the largest organ of the body. For an average adult, the skin occupies a surface area of approximately 3,000 square inches. It covers the body and protects the underlying tissues from bacterial invasion, from drying out and from harmful light rays. In addition to its protective function, the skin helps to control the temperature of the body, prevents excessive loss of inorganic and organic materials, receives stimuli from the environment, stores chemical compounds, excretes water and salts, and synthesizes several important compounds.

Structurally, the skin consists of two principal parts. The outer, thinner portion, which is composed of cells known as epithelium, is called the epidermis. The epidermis is cemented to the inner, thicker, connective tissue part, which is called the dermis. Beneath the dermis is a subcutaneous layer of tissues. The combining form *sub* means under. The subcutaneous layer is also known as the superficial fascia, and it consists of areolar and adipose tissues. Fibers from the dermis extend down into the superficial fascia and anchor the skin to the subcutaneous layer. The superficial fascia, in turn, is firmly attached to underlying tissues and organs.

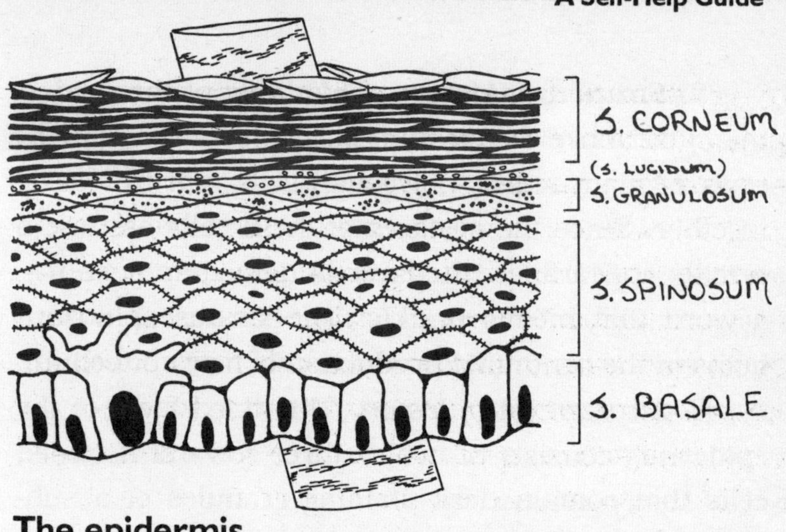

The epidermis

The epidermis is composed of stratified epithelium in four or five cell layers, depending on its location on the body. In areas where exposure to friction is greatest, such as the palms of the hands and soles of the feet, the epidermis has five layers. In all other parts of the body, the epidermis has four layers. The names of these layers from the inside outward are as follows:

1. *Stratum basale.* This is a single layer of columnar cells capable of continuous cell division. The epidermis grows by the division of cells in the stratum basale and deep layers of the stratum spinosum, the next higher layer. As these cells multiply, they push up toward the surface. Their nuclei degenerate, and these cells then die. Eventually, these cells are shed in the top layer of the epidermis.

2. *Stratum spinosum.* This layer of the epidermis, just above the stratum basale, contains 8 to 10 rows of many-sided (polygonal) cells that fit closely together. Since the surfaces of these cells assume a prickly appearance, the layer is named spinosum—a word that means prickly. The stratus spinosum helps in the continued production of new epithelium.

3. *Stratum granulosum.* This third layer of the epidermis consists of two or three rows of flattened cells that contain dark staining granules of a substance called keratohyaline. This compound is involved in the first step of keratin formation. Keratin is a waterproofing protein found in the top layer of the epidermis. The stratum granulosum contains cells whose nuclei are in various stages of degeneration. As the nuclei break down, the cells are no longer capable of carrying out vital metabolic reactions, and they also die.

4. *Stratum lucidum.* This layer exists only in the thick skin of the palms of the hands and the soles of the feet. It consists of three or four rows of clear, flat, dead cells that contain droplets of a translucent substance called eleidin. Eleidin is formed from the keratohyaline and is eventually transformed to keratin. This layer is so named because of the translucent property of eleidin. The word *lucidus* means clear.

5. *Stratum corneum.* This layer consists of twenty-five to thirty rows of flat, dead cells containing the protein keratin. The keratin serves as a waterproof covering. These cells are continuously shed and replaced. The stratum corneum serves as an effective barrier against light and heat waves, bacteria, and many chemicals.

The color of the skin is due to a yellow to black pigment called melanin. This pigment is found throughout the basale and spinosum layers and in the granulosum of all caucasian people. In blacks, melanin is found in all epidermal layers. When the skin is exposed to ultraviolet radiation, both the amount and darkness of melanin increase, which causes tanning and further protects the body against radiation. Thus, melanin serves a very important protective function. Another pigment called carotene is found in the corneum and fatty areas of the dermis in oriental people. Together, carotene and melanin account for the yellowish hue of their skins. The pink color of caucasian skin is due to blood vessels in the dermis. The redness of the vessels is not heavily masked by the pigment. The epidermis has no blood vessels.

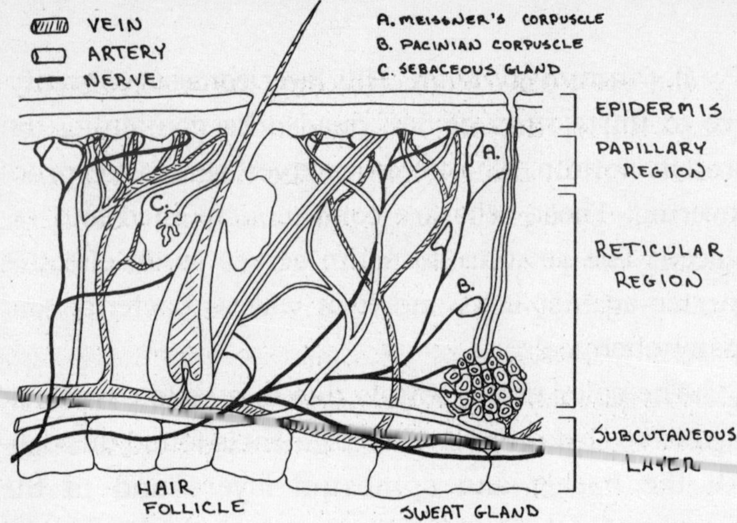

The dermis

The second principal part of the skin, the dermis, is composed of connective tissue containing collagenous and elastic fibers. Numerous blood vessels, nerves, glands and hair follicles are also embedded in the dermis. The upper region of the dermis, which is about one-fifth of the total layer, is referred to as the papillary region. This part of the dermis is so named because its surface area is greatly increased by small, finger-like projections called papillae. These structures project into the epidermis and contain loops of capillaries. In some cases, the papillae contain Meissner's corpuscles, which are nerve endings that are sensitive to touch. The dermis also contains nerve endings called Pacinian corpuscles, which are sensitive to deep pressure, a slightly different response to touch.

The series of ridges marking the external surface of the epidermis are caused by the size and arrangement of the papillae in the dermis. Some of the ridges cross at various angles and can be seen on the back surface of your hand. Other ridges on the palms and fingertips prevent slipping. The ridge patterns on the tips of the fingers and thumbs are different in each individual. Because of this, fingerprints can be taken and accurately used for purposes of identification.

The remaining portion of the dermis is called the reticular region. This area of the dermis contains many blood vessels and also contains collagenous and elastic fibers. The spaces between the interfacing fibers are occupied by adipose tissue and sweat glands. The reticular zone is attached to the organs beneath it, such as bone and muscle, by the subcutaneous layer.

It should now be very obvious that the skin, despite its relatively simple physical appearance, is a very complex organ capable of carrying on numerous activities essential to life. The tissues of the skin are joined to form an organ that performs specific activities.

The various epithelial layers of the epidermis protect, waterproof and add new cells, while the connective tissues (areolar and adipose) of the dermis protect, contain nerve endings for touch and pressure, and connect the epidermis to the subcutaneous layer.

Epidermal derivatives

Organs that are derived from the skin, such as hair, glands and nails, perform functions that are necessary and sometimes vital. Hair and nails offer further protection to the body, whereas the sweat glands perform the vital function of helping to regulate body temperature.

Hair

Certain growths of the epidermis variously distributed over the body are hairs and pili. Some of the regions of the body not covered by hair are the surfaces of the palms of the hands and the undersides of the fingers, the back surfaces of the fingers from the second joint to the fingertips, the soles of the feet, the nipples and the lips. The primary function of hair is protection. Though this protective function is limited, hair guards the scalp from mechanical injury and from the injurious rays of the sun. The eyebrows and eyelashes protect the eyes from foreign particles, and the hair in the nostrils and external ear canal also protect these structures from both insects and dust particles.

Glands

Two principal kinds of glands associated with the skin are sebaceous glands and sweat glands. Sebaceous glands, with only few exceptions, are connected to hair follicles. They are multilobed structures connected directly to the follicle by a short duct. These glands are absent in the palms and soles and differ in size and shape in other regions of the body. For example, they are fairly small in most areas of the trunk and extremities but are relatively large in the skin of the face, neck, and upper chest. The sebaceous glands secrete an oily substance called sebum, which is a mixture of fats, cholesterol, proteins and inorganic salts. The functions of the sebaceous glands are to keep the hair from drying and becoming brittle, and to form a protective film that prevents excessive evaporation of water from the skin. The sebum also keeps the skin soft and pliable. When sebaceous glands of the face become enlarged because of accumulated sebum, blackheads are produced. Since sebum is fine food for certain bacteria, this frequently results in pimples or boils.

Sweat (sudoriferous) glands are distributed throughout the skin except on the nail beds of the fingers and toes, margins of the lips, eardrum, and tip of the penis. In contrast to sebaceous glands, sweat glands are most numerous in the skin of the palms and the soles. They are also found in abundance in the armpits and the forehead. Each gland consists of a coiled end embedded in the subcutaneous tissue and a single tube that projects upward through the dermis and epidermis. This tube, actually an excretory duct, terminates in a pore at the surface of the epidermis. The base of each sweat gland is surrounded by a network of small blood vessels.

Perspiration, or sweat, is the substance produced by sweat glands. It is a mixture of water, salts, urea, uric acid, amino acids, ammonia, sugar, lactic acid, and ascorbic acid. Although perspiration helps eliminate waste materials from the body, its principal value is to help regulate body temperature.

Nails

Modified horny cells of the epidermis are the nails. The cells form a clear, solid covering over the back surfaces of the terminal portions of the fingers. Structurally, each nail consists of a body, root, and lunule. The body is the visible portion of the nail, and the root is hidden under the skin. The lunule is the white half-moon-shaped area at the base of the nail that is the actively growing region. The nails appear pink, except at the lunule, because of the underlying capillaries. These capillaries do not show through the lunule.

Just as the epidermis and dermis form the organ called the skin, the skin together with the accessory organs of hair, glands and nails make up a system called the integumentary system. As a system, the skin and its accessory organs protect underlying tissues from physical injury, harmful light rays, bacterial invasion, and drying out. The system receives stimuli from the environment, eliminates water and salts in the form of perspiration, and helps regulate body temperature. This last function is vital to survival and is a homeostatic (balancing) mechanism.

Psoriatic skin

The epidermal layer on someone with psoriasis is much thicker than that of normal skin and the outer layers of this epidermis do not consist of dead cells. In normal skin the epidermal skin cells mature into flat, thickened "cornified" layer which sloughs off daily. Most of these psoriatic cells are still alive and continuing to grow. This occurs because these cells have moved through to the epidermal layer so quickly that there has not been sufficient time for them to die off. There are also more blood vessels in the upper portion of the dermis and many more cells are found there. These additional cells are white blood cells and they always appear wherever there is inflammation or redness of the skin. These cells travel into the epidermis and form into small clumps, which appear to be tiny pockets of pus, although they are not. This thicker epidermis is the cause of the scaling, and the scales appear to have a silvery appearance because of air spaces between the cells. The increased blood vessels cause the psoriatic patch to be redder in appearance than the surrounding tissue. When the apparently normal appearing skin of individuals with psoriasis (between the patches or elsewhere on the body) is examined under a microscope, it is found to be growing this epidermal layer much more rapidly than that of non-psoriatic individuals.

Skin creases and folds

When the skin folds over on itself, such as the armpits, between the buttocks and the groin or, in the case of obese individuals, under the breasts, across the abdomen and behind the knees, a warm moist area of skin exists. In these areas the psoriasis often does not produce scaling, but has a red fleshy appearance. It does appear to be sore although usually it is not. The skin in these areas is more sensitive than other places and the treatment needs to be gentle. It is often necessary to use a steroid cream which can be combined with a weak tar cream. To add to the problem, this type of psoriasis seems to be more resistant to treatment and may remain long after other patches have been resolved. Anything that the individual can do which will reduce areas of skin folds, such as losing weight, will decrease the occurrence of psoriasis in these areas.

Scalp psoriasis

Half of the people who have psoriasis have it on their scalp. Excessive scaling together with inflammation and length of the hair on the head can make this condition difficult to treat. The scales tend to stick together more tightly in this area and form thick, soft crusts and are very itchy. Many sufferers worry that they will lose their hair with the condition but, in fact, that is most unusual. Psoriasis only affects the skin in the upper portion of the hair follicle and not in the deeper part, where the root of the hair bulb is located. Anyone who is losing their hair and has psoriasis probably has another condition such as male pattern baldness (which also affects women) that should be discussed with the physician.

Several other scalp conditions appear to be psoriasis, such as seborrheic dermitis or seborrheic eczema, so a correct diagnosis is absolutely necessary as the treatments for these two conditions are quite different than that for psoriasis.

The most effective treatments for psoriasis of the scalp are messy and smelly ointments which contain strong coal tar, adding to the problem of treating the scalp and preserving the appearance of the hair at the same time.

Nail psoriasis

Almost fifty percent of individuals with psoriasis and as many as eighty percent of those with psoriatic arthritis find that their nails are affected. There are changes in both the appearance and texture of the fingernails (more frequently than in the toenails) and some individuals have the psoriasis in this location only.

In severe cases of nail psoriasis it is possible to be disabled because of the difficulty in using the hands.

The nails lose their normal healthy appearance and become yellowed or discolored. The most frequent symptom of the condition is the appearance of pits or shallow depressions on the nail itself. These depressions are usually less than one millimeter in diameter. Sometimes the nails are furrowed, with depressions and/or grooves, giving the nail an irregular surface and rough appearance. Occasionally the nail becomes detached from the nail bed--a condition called onycholysis. Nail detachment begins at the edge of the nail and may continue backward under the nail until it is completely loosened from the nail bed. Because of the irregular surface and the softness, it is possible to find that these nails frequently have a bacterial or fungal infection in their surface, which results in painful swelling of the skin surrounding the nail.

When the individual is being treated for psoriasis elsewhere, the nails improve at the same time. However, nail psoriasis is difficult to treat. The abnormality of the nail comes from the nail bed where the nail itself is produced (underneath the nail and under the skin between the nail and the nearest finger joint). Any treatment must get through many layers of skin and nail to be effective and for this reason creams and ointments do not penetrate readily. The only really helpful treatment appears to be PUVA.

5

Who gets psoriasis?

The National Psoriasis Foundation reports that psoriasis affects 5 million people in the United States, men and women equally. Between 150,000 and 260,000 new cases occur each year. The annual outpatient cost for treating psoriasis is currently estimated at $1.6 billion to $3.2 billion, with 2.4 million visits to dermatologists yearly.

The average age at onset is 22.5 years, although psoriasis has been known to occur at birth and as late as age 90, while between 10 and 15% of those who get psoriasis are under age 10.

An estimated 400 individuals die from psoriasis-related causes yearly and another 400 are granted disability by the Social Security Administration because of the disease.

Mark Everett, head of the Department of Dermatology at the University of Oklahoma Health Sciences Center, notes that psoriasis occurs in all segments of the population--there does not appear to be any ethnic group which is immune to the apparently inherited condition.

Is psoriasis contagious?

It is not possible to infect others with this skin condition or contract it from someone else. Friends, family or co-workers often worry unnecessarily about contagion and it is in the individual's best interest to see to it that others' concerns are answered to avoid difficulties with uninformed individuals.

All dermatologists will provide the patient with a letter stating that this condition is not infectious, which may relieve the concerns of employers and co-workers.

Do children get psoriasis?

Psoriasis does appear at birth and ten to 15 percent of all individuals with the condition find that it appeared before the age of ten, 30 percent before the age of 20. More girls than boys get the disease in childhood, although the ratio between the sexes in adults is about even.

The disease in childhood is often preceded by some kind of upper respiratory infection, or strep throat. These children should be under the care of a pediatrician for the infection, with a dermatologist undertaking the care of the skin.

Children very frequently have seborrheic psoriasis and scalp psoriasis and frequently infants have plaques in the diaper rash areas of the body. Children with this condition often have a problem with cradle cap (an extensive, thick, greasy scaling of the scalp in the very young). Babies with the condition develop a very angry appearing rash in the diaper area and other skin creases, such as the neck and armpits.

This psoriasis can be treated with gentle moisturizers (such as vaseline-type products) and mild coal tar, after diagnosis. Usually the pediatrician will refer the parents to a dermatologist for an accurate diagnosis if the child continuously has diaper rash which is not healed with routine methods, particularly if there is a history of psoriasis in the family.

Because other children can be cruel to those whose appearance is different, parents can do a lot to support the child with psoriasis.

Understanding and support from parents who take the time to educate themselves will assist the child to live with the discomforts and inconveniences of the disease.

Inquire whether or not other children are teasing or treating the child badly. Discuss the condition with the child's teacher to be certain that he or she understands that the condition is not contagious, and is knowledgeable enough to explain it to other class members who might be picking on the child because of the appearance of the skin.

It is important that the parents set a good example. If one of the parents has the condition, then he or she must demonstrate proper skin and health care. When others ask questions about the condition, answering without shame and embarrassment will aid the child to accept the condition in a matter-of-fact manner.

Because treatments can be time consuming and might become a chore, particularly for a young child, it is best to attempt to make the treatments a pleasant condition. Use this time to give the child full attention, listen to the complaints and remain sympathetic but positive that the treatments will be beneficial.

The National Psoriasis Foundation has a 10-minute video called *Kids With Psoriasis Need Friends Too.* This video is for kindergarten through third grade and can be rented or purchased.

The Foundation also has a pen pal network for children through which a child can correspond with someone else who has the condition.

Does pregnancy affect psoriasis?

Psoriasis sometimes goes into remission during pregnancy; other women have a flare-up during pregnancy. The condition does not affect fertility or the ability to have children. It is possible to pass on the genes for psoriasis, but researchers believe that the genetic code for the condition is so complex that it should not affect the decision to become a parent.

According to a survey conducted by Stanford University doctors, about 40 percent of women who have psoriasis experience an improvement in their condition during their pregnancy. Efforts to duplicate the conditions of pregnancy in nonpregnant women who suffer from psoriasis have, to date, been unsuccessful.

However, women should discuss pregnancy with their physician because there has been some concern reported in the medical journals concerning those who are taking steroids for their condition which can be excreted in breast milk, possibly adversely affect the nursing child.

Heredity

Psoriasis is believed to be an inherited disorder and it has been shown that the tendency to get psoriasis runs in families, although sometimes it skips generations. Approximately one-third of individuals with the condition will have another family member who also has the disease.

In investigations with identical twins (who are identical in their genetic makeup), approximately seventy percent will both be affected, whereas the percentage drops to twenty in fraternal twins.

The frequency of psoriasis is approximately two percent throughout the world--demonstrating that it is a very common skin disorder. It is rare for the condition to begin before age three. The majority, approximately two-thirds, occurs before age thirty. Another fifth of this population will have their first occurrence before age fifty, but after fifty only a very few will develop the disease.

Infection

For those who have this condition, several factors appear to contribute to its appearance. The first is infection. In particular, *Streptococcus bacterium* appears to influence guttate psoriasis and may be important for other types of psoriasis. The fact that infections appear to play a role in the development of the condition brings into question the possibility that the immune system may also be involved.

Medications

It is definitely known that certain medications aggravate the condition, including one common one prescribed for high blood pressure.

Beta-blockers are the most frequently prescribed medications for high blood pressure and heart disease. In additional to helping control these conditions, beta-blockers produce a lot of side effects, which are sometimes severe enough to warrant discontinuance of the drug. One of the most troublesome is a skin reaction typical of psoriasis. Those who had psoriasis previously, even if only mildly, are almost certain to have a dramatic flare-up after starting on a beta-blocker. *The British Medical Journal* reports that fortunately, psoriasis brought on by a beta-blocker normally disappears soon after the drug is discontinued, and other medicines can usually be found to take its place.

Similar psoriasic reactions can occur with the non-steroidal anti-inflammatory drugs (NSAIDs) that are widely used for arthritis and all sorts of aches and pains.

Stress

It is most important to recognize that stress is absolutely a part of the aggravation of psoriasis. "There is overwhelming evidence that stress can trigger psoriasis," says Eugene Farber, MD, president of the Psoriasis Research Institute. Stress can take many different forms and the amount of stress as well as the kind of stress varies greatly from person to person.

Stressors such as life changes appear to be important initiating factors. It is known that stress can influence the skin in many differing ways. The nervous system tells skin cells how fast to grow and when to stop. Stress also influences hormones circulating in the bloodstream, such as adrenaline and steroids.

Once you understand that stress is the most important trigger for an outbreak of psoriasis, you have begun to gain control over the condition.

Diet

Because the condition goes into periodic remissions, it is tempting to think that something in the diet could influence the condition of the skin. To date there are no direct scientific studies that such an effect occurs. However, there are individuals who claim that it does, and for those that find a connection between a particular food and the breakout of plaques, it makes sense to eliminate that food from the diet, if only on a trial basis, to test whether or not the elimination makes any difference in the condition.

Immune system

A recent theory is that there may be an abnormal immune response in the skin which is the origin of psoriasis. It has been suggested that it may be a lack of control of certain cells in the skin that regulate its immune response. This has been suggested because of the promising results obtained with the immune-regulating drug Cyclosporin. Researchers believe that Cyclosporin may actually correct a local change of immunity in the skin.

The new research at the Laboratory for Investigative Dermatology at Rockefeller University in New York, which points to the immune system as the causative factor in the origins of the disease, further bolsters the abnormal immune response theory.

The human body continually attempts to maintain normal health by counteracting various harmful stimuli in the environment. Frequently, these stimuli are disease-producing organisms, known as *pathogens*, or the toxins they produce as a byproduct of their metabolic activity. In general, the body's defenses against disease are grouped into two broad areas: nonspecific and specific. These defenses provide you with your immunity--that is, the ability to overcome the disease-producing effects of certain organisms. Nonspecific defenses represent a wide variety of body reactions against a wide range of pathogens. Specific defense is the production of a specific antibody against a specific pathogen or its toxin.

Nonspecific defenses

The body deals with any of a variety of pathogens with a nonspecific defense. Conducting such defense is a function of the skin, the mucous membranes, phagocytic leukocytes (toxin and foreign particle devouring cells), and reticuloendothelial (a particular type of skin cell that performs a similar function) cells. For example, the secretions of sweat and sebaceous glands are toxic to many germs. The tear glands of the eyes and the glands in the mucous membranes of the nose and mouth produce an enzyme called lysozyme. This enzyme is also capable of destroying many germs. Many of the microbes that are swallowed with food are killed by the acid secretions of the stomach lining. Finally, throughout the respiratory tract, dust particles that carry microbes are trapped in the sticky mucus. Cilia (tiny hair like projections) that line the respiratory tract move the mucus up to the mouth where it may be swallowed or spit out. If microbes penetrate the defenses of the skin and the mucous membranes, the role of the leukocytes and reticuloendothelial cells is to kill the germs by devouring them before they can travel any further.

Specific defenses

Although the nonspecific defenses of the body are generally effective against germs, they cannot fight the battle alone. Nor can they combat all the toxins that are produced by pathogens. The body's second line of defense is a specific defense that involves the production of antibodies. Antibodies are proteins that inactivate materials known as antigens. Antigens are usually proteins themselves. Pathogens and their toxins are examples of antigens. The antigen-antibody response is a very specific defense because only a particular antibody can combat a particular type of antigen.

Antibody formation

The thymus gland's job is to teach cells how to produce antibodies. Many years ago it was noticed that children who were born without a thymus could not effectively fight disease. These children usually died from a serious infection before they were very old. Researchers also observed that if the thymus was removed from a mouse at the time of birth, the animal was unable to produce antigen-antibody responses. If the researchers delayed the removal of the thymus until the mouse was several weeks old, the antigen-antibody response was normal.

During the first several years of a child, the thymus appears to set up the body's antibody system. Certain wandering epithelial cells become trapped in lymph nodes and other organs early in life. These are the cells that become reticuloendothelial cells. Some investigators have suggested that these wandering cells remain in the thymus for some time before they settle down all throughout the body. During this stay, the thymus changes the DNA of these cells so that they are programmed to make antibodies. Once the thymus has programmed the wandering cells, its role is finished.

When a foreign antigen enters the body sometime later in life, it stimulates the antibody-producing cells. These cells then respond by producing the antibodies they have been programmed to make, thus fighting off invaders and keeping us healthy.

Active and passive immunity

Whether or not a germ makes someone sick often depends on whether or not the person has been exposed to it before. The first time a cell is exposed to an antigen, its antibody response is a little slow to start. This is because the cell needs time to make the proper adjustments in its protein manufacturing assembly line. During this time, the microbes are free to multiply and produce toxins and other symptoms of the disease. If the same kind of microbe invades the body again in the future, the cells may still be geared to produce the antibody. In this case, the antigen-antibody response may occur before the germs have a chance to bring on the symptoms of the disease. Such protection against future sickness is called active immunity.

Active immunity may also be acquired through vaccinations with dead pathogens or with very low doses of their toxins. The proteins in the dead pathogens are cable of stimulating antibody production, but the killed germs cannot hurt you. Toxins are given in doses just high enough to stimulate antibody-producing cells to go into action.

Another form of immunity is known as passive immunity. This is when antibodies are injected from an animal or from another person who has previously been exposed to a disease. Examples are the vaccinations that are effective against hepatitis and measles.

Many cells of the body produce antibodies. Both the lymphocytes and the reticuloendothelial cells are capable of this function. These cells and their antibodies circulate freely through the blood and lymph system and can get to an antigen quickly. However, the life span of these cells is too short to provide immunity against future attacks. Long-term immunity is thought to be provided by long-lived cells, such as muscle cells, which are also capable of producing antibodies.

Because it is thought that psoriasis's initial appearance often follows an infection, such as a strep throat, and then further flare-ups follow stressful events, it would appear that an ineffective immune response might be at the core of the disease.

It should be made clear that most individuals with psoriasis do not have any problem with their internal immune system. Any increase or decrease in the body's immune system does influence psoriasis, but most people with psoriasis do not have an immune deficiency. If there is any abnormality in the immune function, it is believed by researchers that it is in the immune system of the skin only, and it is most likely that it only affects the skin. People with psoriasis do not display any evidence of general changes in their body's immunoregulation.

The psychology of the skin

Because the skin--our external covering--is so visible, it is, in effect, the window to our self that we display to the entire world. Many judgments about others are made based on the condition of the skin. For the millions who experience the lesions of psoriasis, this very visible skin condition can become a living nightmare. Most people consider the lesions unsightly, and the result can be that the emotional damage inflicted on those with psoriasis by others can be extremely traumatizing. Visible lesions can cause emotional problems ranging from a lack of confidence to frustration, nervousness, shame, depression and even suicidal tendencies.

Dr. Nelson Lee Novick, MD, associate clinical professor of dermatology at the Mount Sinai School of Medicine in New York City, feels that you are most at risk for stress-related skin disorders if you already have a pre-existing skin problem, such as psoriasis. A particularly stressful weekend with the kids might trigger a flare-up, even if you haven't had a breakout in a couple of years. He believes that stress can aggravate existing skin problems.

A growing number of physicians believe that a number of common skin conditions--such as acne, eczema, hives, and psoriasis--can be made worse or have flare-ups triggered by anxiety. "Mothers who work outside of the home and then come home to deal with the children and the house are frequent sufferers of a number of stress-related skin problems," says Caroline Koblenzer, MD, associate clinical professor of dermatology and psychiatry at the University of Pennsylvania.

"I've been dealing with the stress connection for years, " says Jonathan Wilkin, MD, a dermatologist and former director of dermatology at Ohio State University. "In April my office is full of accountants. In December, I see all the department store clerks who have to deal with a harried, present-buying public. In June, I see the caterers and the florists, who often have more weddings than they can handle. I may not see these people for the rest of the year, but when their particularly stressful time of year is at hand, they end up in my office."

Although research scientists say that skin problems cannot be pinpointed directly to stress, and the relationship is complex, the side effects of stress can be quite harmful. "Poor diet, smoking, drinking and staying up late are terrible for your health in general, but your first organ to register the strain is often the skin," says John Koo, MD, vice chairman of the department of dermatology at the University of California San Francisco Medical Center.

Despite all we have heard about the addictive qualities of nicotine and alcohol, it is perfectly human to reach for them when we are under stress. "Alcohol increases the flow of blood to the skin," explains Thomas Hogarty, MD a dermatologist in Sheridan, Wyoming, who specializes in addiction medicine. "Alcohol is very hard on conditions such as hives, flushing and itching. The alcohol makes the skin feel warmer, which makes itching worse. And, because it reduces inhibitions about scratching, there is an opportunity there to do some real damage."

Nicotine does just the reverse, as does caffeine. They do their dirty work by reducing the supply of blood to the skin, and since it is well known that stress triggers an increase in the use of both nicotine and caffeine, they can intensify and accelerate damage. They both constrict the blood vessels that supply the skin with vital nutrients.

The additional danger of caffeine and caffeinated drinks is that since they reduce the blood flow to the skin, reducing both nutrients and the skin's germ fighting cells, there is often a rebound effect when the user tries to cut back on the caffeine. This rebound effect causes blood to rush to the skin, causing flushing and aggravating itching, a potential for causing further skin damage by scratching.

6

Jennifer's story continues

Jennifer tried a lot of things. She changed soaps, she changed cosmetics, she changed shampoos, she wore only cotton. Nothing seemed to make any difference. She began wearing long sleeved blouses and pants. The little short skirts and sleeveless clothing currently in favor with her classmates were relegated to the back of her closet. Cheerleading practice became a living nightmare instead of the fun it had been. Instead of looking forward to practice, Jennifer began to make excuses to avoid going. The most popular girl in the class began to turn down invitations to go anywhere--especially if it involved dressing in a way that would expose her elbows or her knees.

"A swim party?," Jennifer rolled her eyes heavenward and covered the mouthpiece of the phone with her hand. "Give me an excuse, quick," she said to her mother. A litany of excuses began to roll easily off her tongue at any invitation.

"I realize now I was in denial. I had completely rejected the diagnosis of psoriasis. I just wanted it to be something simple, something that I could take care of easily with a face cream or a lotion of some kind. I simply couldn't accept that I had a chronic skin condition that was going to affect me for the rest of my life," exclaimed Jennifer. "You cannot believe how cruel people can be, even complete strangers. I've been asked, 'What's wrong with your skin? Do you have something contagious? Ugh! what is that all over your arms, it looks awful!' People have moved away from me at lunch, and girlfriends who used to trade clothing and hats and stuff like that--well, you can forget about that ever happening again. They just quit making excuses, they tell me they don't want to wear anything I've had on, even though I have explained it isn't contagious."

When Jennifer was asked, and not very kindly either, to give up her place on the cheerleading squad because of the way her knees looked, her real depression began. "I had given up getting up in the morning and looking myself all over in the morning, hoping that I would find that this 'thing' would have mysteriously disappeared overnight. I wanted to find it was all just a bad dream. I stayed home, I wouldn't go to class or anyplace. I wouldn't even go out with my parents, who were more understanding than any of my so-called friends. I just sat around the house in an old grubby warm-up suit and watched TV. Then, my parents began yelling at me, I guess because they were really getting worried, and I didn't care at all; I figured my life was ruined, so what was the difference, let them yell. My parents talked to me about courage, courage to face discrimination and know I was a worth-while person. They talked about having self-respect and self-esteem and the courage to deal with my problems. At that time I didn't understand what they were talking about. They suggested that I read a couple of books, one was John Updike's book, *At War With My Skin.* Even after I reluctantly read it, I didn't get the meaning for me. It wasn't till some years later that I understood what my father was talking about; but . . . more of that later. Then my father suggested that we find another doctor, go to a specialist, a dermatologist. That was the next step."

Getting the right diagnosis

Many general practitioners or family practice doctors are the first to see individuals when they first experience psoriasis. Frequently these doctors are unfamiliar with the differing types of psoriasis, or they might make an inappropriate diagnosis and provide an inappropriate treatment.

Once you suspect you might have psoriasis, it is best to be seen by a dermatologist, a doctor who specializes in treating the skin. The dermatologist may suggest a skin biopsy to be absolutely sure of the diagnosis. This is a relatively painless procedure. First the skin is numbed by a local anesthetic and a small sample of skin is removed, which is then examined under a microscope. The microscopic sample will reveal certain characteristics of the tissue cells of psoriasis which cannot be seen by a superficial examination of the skin. Once a skin biopsy has been performed and a definite diagnosis made, the dermatologist can then formulate a treatment plan specific to the individual.

A dermatologist has many resources available for the treatment of psoriasis, including the knowledge of where you can go for more sophisticated facilities and treatment, should that be necessary. With the assistance of a dermatologist, it is possible that the disease can improve to the fullest extent and can clear for lengthy periods with the proper use of differing treatments, when appropriate. With the knowledge that lengthy remissions are possible, the impact of the condition on the patient can be reduced greatly.

Because psoriatic arthritis affects approximately ten percent of all the individuals with psoriasis, the dermatologist may recommend a rheumatologist who will handle the treatment of someone with this type of arthritis.

What is psoriatic arthritis?

This form of psoriasis affects approximately 10 percent of all individuals with the disease. It is most common in the hands and the feet, and is characterized by the presence of the B27 antigen in a large number of patients. Rheumatoid arthritis and psoriasis are two separate diseases that may coexist. Psoriatic arthritis, however, is a different disease with its own identifiable characteristics. It can also cause inflammation, swelling and pain of the larger joints of the body, including the elbows, knees, hips and the spine. As in all arthritis, psoriatic arthritis causes stiffness, pain and decreased movement in all the joints it affects.

Both adults and children can have this type of arthritis. In approximately 85 percent of adults who have this condition, psoriasis precedes the onset of the arthritis, sometimes for several decades. The skin and joints become afflicted at the same time in about 10 percent of the cases, with psoriasis of the nails appearing as part of the condition.

Just the opposite is true in children, with the arthritis preceding the psoriasis in approximately 50 percent of the cases, and girls appear to have psoriatic arthritis approximately three times more frequently than boys.

There are two rare types of arthritis which seem to appear almost exclusively in people with psoriasis. One is destructive of the bones and joints (particularly of the hands and feet) which can result in the shortening of the fingers and toes, in a sausage-like deformity, which is quite disabling. In the other, asymmetric involvement of large and small joints including the sacroiliac and the spine is common. The antigen HLA B27 is often present in these patients. This psoriatic arthritis occasionally affects the bones of the pelvis.

Whether or not psoriasis and arthritis are involved together, the arthritis is treated in the same way as in individuals who do not have attendant psoriasis. Treatment entails taking aspirin or other anti-inflammatory drugs. Steroid injections may offer temporary improvement. In the more severe cases, injectable gold is helpful and usually produces results as good as those achieved in rheumatoid arthritis.

At present, researchers are studying the link between arthritis and psoriasis. One group of researchers has found that individuals with severe psoriasis of the skin appear to have a greater tendency to get arthritis, and another study indicates that individuals with pustular psoriasis were more likely to develop psoriatic arthritis.

Asymmetric arthritis

70 percent of psoriatic arthritis is asymmetric. Two or three joints are usually involved on either the toes or the fingers. The swelling that is apparent is known as sausage digit, because of the appearance of the toes or fingers involved. Although mostly in these areas, it may also involve the wrists, elbows, ankles or knees.

Symmetric polyarthritis

This type occurs in as many as fifteen percent of individuals, and is quite similar to simple rheumatoid arthritis. Both X-rays and blood tests are used by rheumatologists to determine whether the disease is rheumatoid arthritis or psoriatic arthritis. The disease occurs far more frequently in women than in men.

Deforming polyarthritis

Five percent of all individuals with the disease have this severe form. It is characterized by sausage digits (as described above) and quite severe deformities of the toes.

Spondylitis with or without sacroliitis

Spondylitis is an inflammation of the spine, which can be especially severe at the sacroiliac (sacroilitis).

Five percent of individuals with the disease have this condition. It sometimes occurs simultaneously with other kinds of psoriatic arthritis. In the early stages it is characterized by lower back pain and stiffness. Sometimes individuals may develop a severe loss of mobility in the spine.

What is Koebner phenomenon?

Koebner phenomenon is a diagnostic feature of psoriasis. When there is trauma to the skin, a new psoriasic plaque quite frequently will appear at the site. Thus, scratches or surgical incisions elicit linear lesions that should alert the physician to the diagnosis of psoriasis.

What is seborrheic dermitis?

Seborrheic dermitis is a condition which affects the seborrheic areas of the skin (the glands which secrete a greasy lubricating substance). These are areas of the face around the creases of the nose, the eyebrows, scalp and the borders of the hairline. Other parts of the body may be affected, including the armpits, groin and the front of the chest. The condition looks red, and slightly scaly and itchy. It is often seen as severe dandruff.

Mild seborrheic dermitis is fairly common and often individuals with the more severe type of the condition also have psoriasis at the same time. It is generally believed that there is a common genetic disorder which may lead to the development of seborrhea, psoriasis, or both.

Seborrheic dermitis is often related to an excess of yeast on the skin. Common skin yeast lives on flaking dead skin scales of most people, but in individuals prone to seborrheic dermitis it is more pervasive. This condition should be diagnosed by a dermatologist and treated with a yeasticide because it needs to be treated, along with the psoriasis, in order to clear the skin.

What is pityriasis rubra pilaris?

While not psoriasis, this is a skin disease that appears to be genetically determined, with onset in infancy or childhood, or as an acquired disease which appears during the fourth to sixth decades. In either form the involved skin will have a diffuse salmon color with sharply bordered areas of normal skin (known as island sparing); a waxy, yellow skin on the palms of the hands and soles of the feet which is similar to carnuba wax in appearance; reddened papules of the lower surfaces of the fingers and toes.

The condition may resolve itself spontaneously in two to four years in approximately 80 percent of the patients. It is quite difficult to differentiate from psoriasis and, for this reason, an accurate diagnosis is important. The primary treatment is with etretinate.

What is eczema?

Another skin condition, dermatitis, or eczema is a superficial inflammation of the skin which is characterized by vesicles, redness, swelling, oozing, crusting, scaling, and usually, itching.

Contact dermatitis, or eczema, is an acute or chronic inflammation, produced by substances which come in contact with the skin. Common examples are strong alkalis, acids, solvents, soaps, and detergents. Patients often find it difficult to believe that they have become allergic to substances they have used for years or to medications used to treat their dermitis, but the ingredients in topical medications constitute a major cause of allergic contact dermatitis; antibiotics, antihistamines, anesthetics, antiseptics, are examples of products that can become cause for contact dermatitis. Other commonly implicated substances include plants (poison ivy, oak and sumac, ragweed, primrose); many potential sensitizers used in manufacturing (tanning agents and dyes, rubber in bras and other wearing apparel); metal compounds (chrome and nickel); cosmetics (nail polish, deodorants). The symptoms can range from a transient redness to severe swelling and itching. The treatment is the removal of the offending agent.

Atopic dermitis or eczema is a chronic, itching and superficial inflammation of the skin which can occur in a person with a personal or family history of allergic disorders (e.g., hay fever, asthma). The cause is unknown but frequently, numerous inhalants and foods will produce the redness and itching reaction. Again, removal of the offending agent is the treatment. Corticosteroid creams are the most effective medication.

It is quite obvious that eczema is very different from psoriasis but for those who are unfamiliar with either condition, it is easy to understand how one skin condition can look very much like another.

7

Life with psoriasis

Once you have a definite diagnosis of psoriasis, it is best to follow your doctor's instructions, including the taking of specific medications. However, there are a number of things you can do to make yourself more comfortable. As you know, psoriasis is a disease of remissions, which means that there will be times when you are clear of the outbreaks. During these times it is easy to forget that you have this condition, and get careless about the care of your skin. Taking the time in everyday living to do the things that keep your skin soft, supple and intact can go a long way toward making living with the condition easier.

What are the treatments for psoriasis?

At the present time, there is no cure for psoriasis--but that doesn't mean you should just give up and live with it. There are a great many medications, treatments and life style changes which can greatly enhance the comfort level of someone with the disease, which can heal the skin and cause psoriasis to go into remission. Periodic remissions can relieve the individual of lesions for times as long as a year or more.

Treatments are aimed at temporarily clearing the plaques or significantly improving the appearance of the skin. The goal at the present is to clear the lesions from the skin. Once a treatment accomplishes this goal, the medication is temporarily discontinued and then resumed when another flare-up occurs.

The type of treatment your doctor will prescribe for you will depend on several factors: the type of psoriasis, its location on the body, its severity, your age and medical history. Medications which require a doctor's prescription need to be followed precisely. It is a mistake to use the medication prescribed for someone else (and this is tempting if someone else in the family has psoriasis) as each individual case is different and may require different treatment at differing times in the course of a flare.

Topical medications are used for mild to moderate psoriasis. These treatments include emollients (moisturizers), steroids (cortisone-type medications), anthralin, various coal tar preparations and vitamin D3. These may be used alone, in combination, or with ultraviolet light (UVB). Sunbathing is sometimes sufficient to clear psoriasis for some individuals because of the exposure to natural ultraviolet light.

Treatments for moderate to severe psoriasis can include the above listed topical medications, ultraviolet light type B (UVB); PUVA (an oral or topical medication, plus ultraviolet light type A); an oral or injectable methotrexate (MTX); and oral retinoid medications (Tegison and Accutane). These may be used alone or in a combination specifically for your condition. Systemic treatments for severe psoriasis are more toxic than topical treatments and their benefits must be weighed against the risk entailed.

A practical rule in psoriasis therapy is to use the most effective treatment for the individual that poses the least amount of risk from side effects. Generally, the doctor will begin with the least potent therapy and work up until one is found that will clear the plaques for that individual person.

There appears to be no single treatment that works for everyone. Reactions to treatments vary from individual to individual and sometimes experimentation is required before an effective approach is found.

Treatment regimens may need periodic adjustment. Sometimes an effective treatment will stop being effective as the patient's body becomes resistant, and that will necessitate a re-evaluation and possibly the recommendation of a different therapy.

Emollients

Emollients are any of the lubricants or moisturizers which will help restore moisture and flexibility to psoriatic skin. They can aid in reducing scaling, itching and inflammation. There are a great many emollients available over-the-counter and it is best to use one regularly. It is suggested that you purchase the smallest container possible to find out if the particular emollient is beneficial, and those with heavy perfumes should be avoided.

The thicker the cream or lotion, the more effective the emollient is likely to be. They seem to slow the loss of water through the skin layers from bathing and phototherapy treatments. Frequently, the physician will request that the patient apply an emollient just prior to their phototherapy session. Pure petroleum jelly is highly effective.

It is important to use an emollient after bathing, showering or swimming. Application twice a day will provide the greatest benefit. A lighter emollient for daytime use and a heavier, thicker one for nighttime use is suggested. Careful attention to the regular use of the emollient can relieve painful dry skin as well as reduce scaling and inflammation. With some time allowance and planning, use of the emollient will become just another part of your daily routine, like brushing your teeth and combing your hair.

One of the benefits of emollients is that there are no side effects.

Topical steroids

Topical steroids are the most frequently prescribed therapy for the treatment of localized areas of psoriasis. Topical steroids come in various strengths, from very mild to very potent. The higher the strength of the medication, the more effective the medication will be, but the potential side effects also increase.

Steroids are prescription medications. There are very low-strength hydrocortisone preparations which can be purchased over-the-counter but they have not been found to be very useful in the treatment of psoriasis.

Steroids are not usually effective in producing remissions in severe psoriasis, and can result in a rebound (that is, the condition can come back as bad or worse than before the treatment) of the disorder if used in large portions. Many patients misuse this prescription medication, thinking that if a little is good, more would be better. Steroids should be used sparingly and applied only to the areas directed. They should not be applied to healthy skin areas and should not be used in areas where there are other lesions for which the dermatologist has prescribed some other medication.

Topical steroids come in ointments, creams, lotions, aerosols or tapes. The dermatologist will recommend which type and potency are proper for your condition, and how frequently you should use a steroid.

Thick, plaque-type psoriasis on the elbows, palms of the hands, knees, soles of the feet and other thickly skinned areas tend to resist the absorption of steroids and frequently require one of the higher strength prescriptions. Lesions in body folds, the groin, eyelids and other areas where the skin is thin are usually more sensitive to steroid treatment with the result that it is more effective in these areas.

Topical steroids should not be used after the condition has cleared, because steroids thin out the skin. Thinning the skin is the result you are looking for in the thick, plaque-type lesions, but extremely thin skin is subject to breaks in its integrity which can result in openings for other infections. Thinning of the skin as a side effect can be a particular problem, particularly for young children and babies, as their skin is naturally thinner than that of an adult.

Other side effects include acne, rosacea, dermitis and secondary infections of the skin. Glaucoma can result from the use of topical steroids close to the eyes.

Systemic (internal) steroids

Systemically administered steroids (internally administered steroid medication--pill or muscular injection) are generally avoided in the treatment of psoriasis because of the potential for serious side effects. Occasionally a small dose of an oral steroid (such as prednisone) may be given for a brief time to control a sudden flare and its use is carefully monitored by the physician because systemic steroids can also cause psoriasis to worsen, and precipitate life-threatening pustular forms of psoriasis.

Injected intra-lesional steroids

Sometimes the dermatologist will inject steroid medication directly into an isolated lesion (a plaque) because it can be effective in clearing the lesion and seldom produces side effects.

Occlusion

Several studies indicate that covering psoriasis lesions with a tape dressing, plastic wrap, or a special suit for days and sometimes weeks is effective, particularly when used in conjunction with topical steroid medications. A shower cap or a wrap of plastic wrap over the head can be effective for scalp psoriasis. This treatment appears to be effective only for small areas and if the area gets too moist and then becomes infected the psoriasis can get worse.

Extensive psoriasis on the body and the limbs can be occluded with a special suit that is worn to enhance the effects of medications.

Coal tar

Crude coal or coal tar solutions are often used in treatment of psoriasis. They come in both prescription or over-the-counter medications.

Almost fifty years ago, Dr. Goeckerman of the Mayo Clinic invented this therapy, which can be both messy and time consuming but quite effective.

Tar for the body is applied directly to the affected area or it can be added to bath water as a form of a soak. It can also be used in combination with topical steroids.

Tar is sometimes used in combination with ultraviolet light, type B (UVB). When administered in this form, it is left on the involved skin for a considerable period of time, ranging from a couple of hours to overnight, prior to exposure to UVB light. The tar is then removed from the skin prior to the exposure.

There are different types of tars used (shale, wood and coal) but coal seems to be the most effective.

The physician will determine the regime that is best for the patient. Frequently a topical steroid is applied to lesions once or twice a day and then the tar preparation is applied at night before retiring.

One of the problems with the tar is that it is messy. It can stain everything that comes in contact with it--furniture and clothing. It is best to apply it and then wait fifteen minutes before dressing or retiring to allow most to be absorbed into the skin. Older clothing or clothing and bedding that is already stained is the best to use at this time. Some of the purified tar gels, lotions, creams or oils do not stain clothing as readily as the coal tar.

When using tar it is best to avoid exposing the treated skin areas to sunlight as it increases the risk of sunburn.

Anthralin

Anthralin is a topical prescription medication that is a synthetic substance made from anthracene, a coal tar derivative that can be effective in clearing lesions. It is prescribed in differing concentrations in ointment, paste, cream or stick form. The higher strength compounds cause staining of the skin and irritation, and some patients are unable to tolerate even the lower concentrations, which makes it awkward for home use.

Lower-strength anthralin compounds have been developed which have made this therapy more tolerable and can be used on both the body and the scalp. It takes longer to work than steroids, in many cases as long as six weeks.

Anthralin is applied topically to the affected area and is left on for a short period of time, never overnight. It is used in combination with UVB therapy.

One of the difficulties with the use of Anthralin is that it stains everything, except psoriasic skin, including normal skin, clothing, bathtubs, grout, even ceramic shower tiles.

One of the at-home uses of anthralin is to add it to an oil-in-water emulsion which makes it easier to get into the plaques. It is applied using disposable plastic gloves, left in place for 15 to 60 minutes and then washed off with liquid soap and water, finishing up with a moisturizer applied to the treated skin.

Anthralin should not be applied to lesions on the face or groin. It is necessary to keep this product away from the eyes.

Scientists are constantly working on improving these drugs to reduce staining, messiness and irritation. The physician or dermatologist will be aware of any new forms of these treatments as they are introduced and can explain them and decide whether or not they are appropriate for the individual patient.

Vitamin D3

Vitamin D3 or calcipotriene (Dovorex) is a topical medication available for mild to moderate psoriasis. It has few side effects if used as directed, and it is odorless, nonstaining and does not cause skin thinning. Normally, it is applied to lesions twice a day. It should not be used on the face or in the area of the genitals because it can cause irritation, and it is not recommended for children or for use during pregnancy.

Researchers at Japan's Osaka University Medical school obtained promising results with various forms of the active D3, and Michael F. Holick, an endocrinologist of the Boston University School of Medicine obtained FDA approval in 1990 to begin treating patients with D3. Dr. Holick told a reporter, "This is a major therapeutic approach for treating this very difficult skin disease."

Other creams aim at reducing inflammation, but vitamin D3 may actually slow the growth of psoriasis-struck cells that otherwise pile up. The immunologic effects of active D3 analogs may play a role in the immunologic aspects of the disorder. When this cream was tested against the traditional corticosteroid cream in 345 people with psoriasis, the D3 came out on top when it came to reducing the affected areas and severity of the disease. After six weeks of using each cream on different halves of their bodies, 82 percent of the D3-treated sides of these patients had improved greatly or cleared up, while only 69 percent of the corticosteroid-cream sides had the same response.

This form of Vitamin D3 is the hormonal form of the vitamin produced by the kidney, and is not the same as the commercial vitamin supplements that are taken orally. Ingesting large amounts of Vitamin D can have serious side effects.

Keratolytics

Salicylic acid is a keratolytic that helps to remove scales and is often combined with steroids, anthralin and tar to enhance their effectiveness. These clear, non-greasy lotions, creams or gels are easy to use; they remove very thick scales and work with other topical treatments.

Other keratolytic agents are lactic acid and ammonium lactate, and they provide better results when combined with tar preparations than alone.

Ultraviolet light, type B (UVB)

If the psoriasis is quite extensive, ultraviolet light is a good choice for treatment.

The ultraviolet rays of the sun are the most natural treatment for psoriasis available, and nearly eighty percent of people with the condition have observed that they improve in sunny climates. Many individuals have observed that their condition improves in the summer and gets worse in the winter, when there is less sunlight. It is well known that mood may change when the days get shorter. Biochemical and hormonal changes occur in everyone as there is less sunlight and for some individuals this is known as SAD, seasonal affective disorder. For people with this condition, special ultraviolet light therapy is prescribed, but many home ultraviolet machines used for SAD are not powerful enough to do any good on psoriasis. If you should use an ultraviolet home machine, the dermatologist will want to carefully instruct you in the use of these home treatments. You need a full skin examination every three months while conducting home ultraviolet treatment. After therapy is completed, an annual skin evaluation should be made to ensure there are no signs of skin cancer.

There are a variety of home treatment units which vary in intensity of the ultraviolet energy they produce. Your doctor will give you specific directions concerning the length of exposure and times. It is necessary to maintain a constant distance from the lights so that the amount of exposure can be determined with accuracy.

It is necessary to wear UV protective glasses to protect the eyes during treatment.

Many of the light machines come with a timer and that should be set to avoid being burned or overexposed.

You will be requested to have a follow-up visit every three months for a routine skin examination. This is to ascertain whether or not the UV is causing additional skin damage. If you are unable to keep this follow-up appointment you should stop the treatments until your skin can be examined.

It may be that psoriasis that worsens during the winter months may be related to seasonal affective disorder because of the differences that occur with biochemical and hormonal changes.

People who have had skin cancer in addition to psoriasis should be aware that they are at greater risk for developing new skin cancers in any part of the body and should exercise caution about exposing themselves to lengthy sunbathing.

These rays, ultraviolet B, occur naturally in sunlight and it is that spectrum of the sunlight which causes sunburns. Artificial UVB is used to treat a number of other skin disorders as well as psoriasis, such as lichen planus, eczema, fungal infections and certain types of acne.

UVB therapy can produce a temporary clearance in most patients. The length of remission varies among individuals. It can be administered to a particular area of the body or the entire body surface. It can be administered at a center, or home light units can be purchased.

UVB can be used alone, with emollients such as petrolatum, or with over-the-counter or prescription tar preparations. The combination of UVB and tar therapy is known as the Goekerman regimen.

PUVA (Psoralen and ultraviolet light, type A)

Thousands of years ago, the Egyptians treated psoriasis by eating the extract of a weed, Ammi majus, which contains psoralens, and grows along the Nile River, and then exposing the affected area to the sun.

PUVA combines the use of a photosensitizing medication named psoralen and long-wave ultraviolet light, UVA. The patient takes an oral dose of the psoralen prescription medication which makes the skin sensitive to UVA light, and then exposes the involved skin to UVA light.

PUVA is effective in eighty-five to ninety percent of patients, and remissions can last as long as a year or more.

Psoralens are drugs that are activated by ultraviolet light and enable the physician to target specific diseased tissues without destroying normal body tissue. Porsalen interacts with molecules on the surface of cells. Francis Gasparro and Richard Edelson of Yale University School of Medicine reported at a photobiology symposium that when they treated human lymphocytes with activated psoralen, it bound to cell membrane DNA. At the same meeting, Jeffrey Laskin, of Robert Wood Johnson Medical School in New Jersey, presented evidence of a cell membrane protein receptor for psoralen. They believe that psoralen normalizes the function of an enzyme important in cell division. Francesco dall'Acqua of the University of Padova in Italy, reported that psoralen applied to rats' skin bound to the lipids of skin cells. Their results may help scientists develop synthetic analogs of psoralen.

It should be noted that Robert Stern, of Harvard Medical School, found that patients who receive this therapy are far more likely than the general population to develop squamous cell carcinoma and basal cell carcinoma, two normally nonfatal skin cancers. Stern recommends that PUVA be alternated with other treatments to lower the risk.

Psoralens are found normally in carrots, celery, parsley, dill, limes, figs and chrysanthemums. Workers such as those in the produce department of an Oregon supermarket recently suffered an outbreak of phytophotodermitis. Doctors concluded that the psoralens on the hands of these workers who routinely trimmed vegetables made them sensitive to ordinary sunlight to such an extent that they developed skin irritation. It was found that they needed to wear gloves at work and avoid sunlamps to prevent the action of the psoralens on their skins, which did not need any such treatment.

Most PUVA ultraviolet lights are broad-spectrum UVA fluorescent lights. This type of light produces significant heat, so most of the treatment centers provide adequate ventilation and air-conditioning, as well as showers, because the user often perspires heavily during the PUVA treatment.

Individuals who are candidates for PUVA phototherapy are only those with incapacitating psoriasis, failure of conventional topical therapy or of tar and ultraviolet phototherapy, or those who have had a rapid relapse after these forms of therapy. Individuals who have previous or present skin cancers, previous x-ray therapy to the skin, or cataracts are not candidates for this treatment.

Treatment will require use of protective glasses on the day of the treatment and during the therapy.

Because the psoralen stays on the skin for approximately eight hours after ingestion, it is necessary to avoid sun exposure after the treatment. Patients are advised to use sunscreen on unprotected areas of skin and to wear garments with long sleeves and long pants.

Twenty percent of all PUVA patients experience occasional nausea and stomach upset; this can be avoided by taking the medication with food or milk.

Methotrexate (MTX)

Methotrexate is a derivative of the same Nile River weed the Egyptians used to treat psoriasis thousands of years ago. It is used in small doses to clear severe and/or disabling psoriasis, and is taken orally or given by injection.

Methotrexate is generally recommended only if other psoriasis therapies have been ineffective or if other therapies cannot be tolerated. It is a potent drug with serious side effects.

Patients with a history of liver disease or who use alcohol excessively cannot use this treatment. When methotrexate is prescribed it is necessary to see the physician every four weeks, and if the treatment is longer than three months, it will be necessary to have a liver biopsy because it can cause serious liver damage. In addition, it has been known to cause birth defects, miscarriage or stillbirth, particularly in the first trimester of a pregnancy. Pregnant women must not take it and women of childbearing years should not become pregnant while using the medication.

The side effects are loss of appetite, nausea,

diarrhea, abnormal liver test results, sores or ulcers inside the mouth. Long-term treatment may result in cirrhosis of the liver.

However, it is the treatment of choice for a number of patients and there are many who tolerate it without any side effects.

Retinoid therapy

Vitamin A derivatives are known as retinoids. Because retinoids are related to Vitamin A, all individuals being treated for psoriasis with one of the oral retinoids should avoid taking vitamin A supplements because they may add to the unwanted side effects of the medication.

Treatment with etretinate (Tegison) is for the most severe, disfiguring, stubbornly resistant psoriasis. It is used with patients who have severe psoriasis and are unresponsive to standard therapies or, for some other reason, cannot use any of the other therapies. It is generally combined with other treatments such as PUVA.

Because etretinate can cause birth defects, women of childbearing years must use effective contraception during treatment with this drug. While Tegison is a potent treatment for psoriasis, it stays in the body for approximately three years and could make pregnancy risky for years to come. It has been shown to be effective in treating erythrodermic psoriasis and pustular psoriasis.

Another form of this medication, acetretin, is currently awaiting FDA approval and it may pose fewer risks to childbearing age women as it clears more rapidly from the body.

Accutane (isotretinoin) is another oral medication sometimes used to control psoriasis. It also has potential birth defect risks, although pregnancy is acceptable once the drug is no longer being used and after an appropriate waiting period.

These drugs have proven to be particularly successful for use with general pustular psoriasis but they have possible side effects such as dryness of the skin, mouth and lips, hair loss, increased fat levels in the blood, altered liver function, and bony overgrowth on the skeleton.

Cyclosporine

Cyclosporine is an immune suppressant used in organ transplantation. It has been found to work very well in treating severe psoriasis. However, it suppresses the body's immune system and its lengthy use may lead to increased risks of cancer.

Cyclosporine is used to bring about a remission, and maintenance therapy is then continued with another treatment deemed appropriate by the physician.

As with all drugs used to treat the patient systemically, it does have potential side effects. It has been associated with kidney damage, and kidney function should be monitored by blood and urine tests throughout the entire time of treatment.

Zonalon

Zonalon is effective in relieving itching. Its active ingredient is the well-known drug Doxepin, which has been used for many years in the treatment of depression. Doxepin also works as an antihistamine, especially when applied directly to the skin, and that is how it relieves itching. Patients apply a thin film of the cream 4 times daily over itching areas of the skin for no more than 8 days, with at least 3-4 hours between applications. Used for too long, too often, or over too large an area of the body's surface, the cream causes drowsiness as the result of the drug being absorbed and getting into the circulation. It has a powerful sedating effect on the nervous system, and it is this effect on the skin's sensory nerves that makes it useful for itching.

Over-the-counter Zostrix

Zostrix cream can be purchased for the relief of itching over-the-counter without a physician's prescription.

A chemical derived from chili peppers, capsaicin causes nerve endings to release a neurotransmitter called substance P which lets the brain know that something painful is going on within the body. Capsaicin can stimulate an increase in the amount of substance P released. Eventually, this can deplete the substance P supply and reduce further releases from the nerve endings.

Knowing that, researchers tried using capsaicin in a cream (brand name Zostrix) to reduce post-operative pain for mastectomy patients and amputees. Further tests found that the cream helped reduce the itching of dialysis patients, the pain from shingles or herpes zoster, and pain and tingling associated with diabetes mellitus.

The cream's pain-relieving success led rheumatologists to wonder if it might help their arthritis patients. In a 12-week study of 113 osteoarthritis patients, 81 percent who regularly rubbed the cream on aching joints had pain reduced by half.

Reducing substance P also helps joints by fighting long-term inflammation. Substance P seems to prolong inflammation. That is bad because if joints stay inflamed, cartilage may break down.

Reporting in the *Journal of the American Academy of Dermatology*, Charles Ellis says that capsaicin can quell the incessant itch associated with psoriasis, possibly shortening outbreaks. Application of the cream depletes the body of substance P that transmits the itch signal to the body. While this is not a cure, it can speed up the healing process by reducing the amount of scratching, which stimulates psoriasis.

Researchers at the University of Michigan medical school found that Zostrix relieved itching in 66 percent of a group of psoriasis patients. The itching in these cases was severe and very troublesome, and had not responded to treatment with cortisone-like steroids. When first applied to the skin, Zostrix causes transitory burning, but the patients in this study did not consider this to be a problem.

One warning: always wash your hands after rubbing on the cream. Should you rub your eyes with the cream on your hands, there is enough capsaicin to make your eyes water and burn.

Treatment of psoriatic arthritis

Anyone who suspects that their condition is psoriatic arthritis in any form should be under the care of a rheumatologist.

Joint stiffness, pain, fatigue and joint swelling all indicate a need for rest. A rheumatologist will recommend a regimen of both rest and mobility-sustaining exercises to maintain the best function of the joints for the individual involved.

Non-steroidal anti-inflammatory drugs can provide relief by reducing inflammation and pain in the joints, but none will provide a remission of the disease--only relief of the symptoms.

It is possible that the physician will prescribe certain drugs to attempt to protect the joints from further destruction, and these should be discussed with the physician managing the particular patient.

None of these medications or treatments are cures, they all reduce the symptoms but . . . you can probably reduce symptoms yourself, by using your doctor-prescribed treatment AND getting control of your stress.

8

Daily living with psoriasis

Living with psoriasis can be difficult. The emotional impact can be devastating. Because the skin is the person's window to the world, the condition is difficult to hide or disguise, and can impair the individual's employability, romantic opportunities, social development and self-esteem.

Treatments can be time consuming and messy.

There are some simple common sense changes that the individual with psoriasis can make that will be helpful to avoid unnecessary problems in day-to-day living.

In some ways the psoriasis sufferer is fortunate. Psoriasis is a stoplight: a warning signal that something in your life needs attention. STOP . . . and take care of both your skin and your stress so that you can be in control.

Clothing

It is perfectly acceptable to cover the affected skin. This helps in preventing the temptation to scratch the itchy plaques, it prevents more irritation, and avoids discomforting questions from insensitive people and strangers concerning the condition. This is especially true for young children who are frequently taunted by classmates. Self-confident adults can handle this kind of questioning or remarks from others; many young children are especially vulnerable to taunts and bullying.

Comfortable fabrics, particularly cotton rather than man-made fibers such as polyester, are less irritating to the skin. Wool next to the skin is known to be irritating even for those who do not have a skin condition. Exposure to sunlight is beneficial, and white, loose-woven cloth will allow some sunlight to pass through to the skin.

There are fabrics now with a special knitting technology that creates tiny pores in the fabric so the sun can penetrate. These fabrics offer up to SPF-20 protection under average natural outdoor tanning conditions. These are available from Comtrad Industries, for men and women, in both bathing suits and shirts.

For more information, contact them at:

Comtrad Industries
2820 Waterford Lake Drive, Suite 106
Midlothian, VA 23113
1-(800)-704-1211

Scalp psoriasis will be less noticeable if dark clothing is avoided, as the flaking scalp scales will be less visible on lighter clothing. If you are using one of the staining shampoos, shampoo the hair away from the face, to prevent the staining material from dripping onto the forehead and into the eyes.

Many of the treatments are ointments and creams which, unfortunately, stain clothing. Older undergarments, already stained, or a special kind of underwear which is known as tubinet and is available from medical supply houses, can prevent valuable clothing from staining by psoriasis treatments. Staining can be lessened by applying treatments at night and then using a moisturizer during the daytime which will reduce flakiness and dryness during the day. Soft, inexpensive cotton undergarments can also be worn under clothing. Inexpensive T-shirts with sleeves can aid in preventing ointments from staining outer garments and they can be disposed of after a few wearings.

Bathing

Everyone's skin is different and everyone's experience with psoriasis is different. Experiment with bathing to see what is best for you. Read the ingredients on the label before selecting soaps, shampoos and bath products. Many of them contain detergents which are drying to the skin as they are meant to dissolve grease. Read the labels for perfumes or bath additives, which may be included to provide lather through a foaming agent, as they are quite often irritants to already sensitive skin. Unless you are employed in an occupation at which you get really dirty (such as garage mechanic or miner), you may want to avoid soap altogether and bathe only with an emollient cream. These creams are also available in lotion form which makes bathing with them easier. Bath oils added to the water or applied to the skin when it is still moist can be beneficial in keeping the skin intact.

Water temperature can affect the way the skin reacts also, so you should experiment with both cool and warm water to see what works best for your particular condition. Baths and heated swimming pools are excellent. They flatten plaques and cut down on scaling, but hot water can make itching worse.

A cold water bath with a cup of apple cider vinegar added is good to decrease itching. Small itching areas can be desensitized by putting some ice cubes in a plastic bag and holding it against the affected area for a few minutes.

After bathing, pat yourself dry--don't rub as this can irritate the skin. Add your moisturizer while the skin is still moist: damp skin helps seal in water.

Shampooing the hair can be difficult when you are using a greasy scalp treatment. It may be beneficial to wear the hair short and wash it lightly more frequently. More frequent washing will also help to keep scaling down. Tar-containing and medicated shampoos can be helpful. Frequently one shampoo which has worked well will stop performing, as the scalp tends to become resistant to the treatment. It is a good idea to change shampoos occasionally and intersperse these treatment shampoos with a mild baby-shampoo formula to avoid this occurring.

Cosmetic hair treatments such as permanent waves and color are acceptable, but remember that they are sometimes harsh to the scalp and should not be done when the scalp or skin at the edge of the hair line is overly sensitive, broken or sore.

Herbalist Jeanne Rose, author of *Jeanne Rose's Herbal Body Book*, recommends taking a soothing bath made with leaves from a healing agent (comfrey root) with a salicylic acid herb like white willow bark.

Care of the nails

When the finger and/or toe nails are affected by psoriasis, they may be thick, with roughened surfaces. They may become yellowed or otherwise discolored, and extensive disease can cause the nails to crumble easily. The nails should be kept short so that pressure will not detach loosened nails. This is best done with a diamond dust nail file rather than attempting to clip or cut them. If the nails have become very thick, it is best to have the clipping done by a chiropodist or podiatrist.

Polishes can be used, but they are difficult to apply or remove from the surface of rough, irregular nails, and, if the nails are badly pitted, polishes only call attention to the condition of the nails rather than protecting them. Read the labels carefully as some of the ingredients in the colored polishes can further destroy the nail, making it more fragile and more brittle.

Wear gloves when working with your hands and avoid activities that might further injure the nails.

Care of skin folds and genitals

Psoriasis in the areas of the armpits, groin, between the buttocks or under pendulous breasts can become extremely uncomfortable. This delicate skin should only be treated with the mildest of creams or ointments and should be kept dry and clean as it is prone to yeast or fungal infections.

When showering, these areas can be washed using the same shampoo that is used for the scalp.

Genital psoriasis may be helped by the use of condoms for men and a lubricating jelly for women to reduce irritation during sexual intercourse.

Housekeeping

Many people with psoriasis are very sensitive to the flakes of dead skin cells they leave behind on furniture, floors and bed sheets. If this is your own home it may be necessary to change the bedding frequently, particularly if a greasy or staining treatment is used. Most family members are understanding of the condition and are not critical of the skin shedding of family members.

If you feel sensitive about staying with relatives or friends, a small portable battery operated vacuum cleaner can be brought along with your luggage so that you can clean up after yourself. In addition, you might bring your own sheets to put down on the bedding so that you do not damage the bed linens of others when you visit.

Care should be taken when using household cleaning products to protect the skin from damage.

Rest

It is important to get adequate rest no matter whether you have a medical condition or not. Fatigue and lack of sleep can add to stress which has already been implicated in triggering psoriasis. It is best to have a regular schedule and a regular bedtime in order to maintain yourself in the best health possible.

Alcohol

Alcohol does not directly affect psoriasis, but there are some treatments that preclude the use of alcohol. Excessive amounts of alcohol can affect all body systems and indirectly undermine overall health.

Nicotine

There does not appear to be any connection to smoking and psoriasis, except for those individuals with pustular psoriasis. Cessation of smoking appears to improve that skin condition dramatically.

Avoid injury

Because flares of psoriasis appear to be related to injured skin, take care in choosing activities. Researchers believe that trauma to the skin may send the skin into an extreme reaction. Be aware of such things as tight shoes, watchbands that rub, dull razors and harsh chemicals, such as those in cleaning and lawn care products.

Weight

It is well-documented that there is a connection between being overweight and psoriasis. It appears to be one of the most reliable connectors. Weight loss has helped many people with the skin condition. Maintaining a normal weight almost always makes psoriasis improve.

Treat infections early

Existing psoriasis is known to worsen when there is an infection present, and it is well-documented that there is a link between infections such as strep throat and the initial onset of psoriasis.

Treat all infections right away and pay extra attention to the psoriasis when you have any type of infection.

Diet

To maintain good health it is important to eat a well balanced diet, with plenty of fresh fruits and vegetables. It is also sensible to eat regular meals, and not skip breakfast or eat a lot of junk foods. If your schedule is busy and you miss meals or grab a quick on-the-run meal, then you are probably contributing to your stress, which is very bad for individuals with psoriasis.

It is apparent that certain foods can promote allergic and/or inflammatory changes in the skin which may be sufficient to trigger a flare.

Supplementation of the diet with vitamins and minerals may be helpful if the diet is inadequate, but it appears that it is quite unnecessary to use macro-amounts of these supplemental nutrients.

There are no scientific studies which have implicated diet in the onset of psoriasis, but there are quite a few people who maintain that adhering to a particular diet or eliminating a particular food from their diets has made a difference.

If you observe that some particular food appears to make a difference in the flares of your psoriasis, it makes sense to keep a food diary to track and then document the evidence of the accuracy of your observation. If, after keeping a food diary for several weeks, you find that there are certain foods you believe contribute to your condition, it would seem prudent to eliminate them from your diet.

Nutritional therapy is a burgeoning area of skin research. Within the past decade, researchers have examined the role of vitamin deficiencies in skin health, prompting some physicians to recommend dietary supplements in some specific cases.

Melvyn Werbach, MD, author of *Healing Through Nutrition*, recommends 3.5 to 5 grams of Vitamin C daily for a three-month trial to help skin conditions. As an antioxidant, Vitamin C is believed to strengthen the immune system.

Zinc may also play a role in keeping skin healthy. According to Werbach, "Because zinc, like Vitamin C, is important for the proper functioning of the immune system, it is not surprising that zinc deficiency appears to be related to a tendency toward recurrent skin infections."

Zinc supplements should only be taken with medical supervision and should not be taken over a long period of time because they may adversely affect cholesterol levels. Werbach recommends a six-week trial period, in which 50 milligrams (mg) zinc with 2 mg copper amino acid chelate is taken three times daily; the dosage of zinc should be reduced once the skin improves.

Recent research has indicated that Omega-6 essential fatty acids may play a role in regulating inflammation and the immune response. (Omega-3 fatty acids may also have these properties, but they are derived from fish oils.) Werbach cites Evening Primrose Oil as a good source of GLA, an Omega-6 fatty acid. An article in the *British Journal of Dermatology* showed Evening Primrose Oil to be particularly effective in alleviating the constant itching caused by rough and thickened skin. Werbach recommends taking 1 to 2 grams of Evening Primrose Oil three times daily for a four-week trial period.

A Swedish study recommends a low-protein, low-fat vegetarian diet.

Cosmetics

Cosmetologist and Hollywood makeup artist Maurice Stein told the editors of *Prevention* magazine that he recommends an over-the-counter cream named *Couvre*, applied with a makeup sponge, that can be applied to the scalp to cover up flaking. He suggests you get the OK from your physician first.

For elbows and knees, he recommends Indian Earth mixed with your emollient and spread over the plaques with a makeup sponge. The emollient will keep the plaques moist, and the Indian Earth will cover their appearance.

Recreation

It does not appear that any recreational activity has any effect on exacerbating psoriasis, so there should be no reason to alter leisure activities. In fact, exercise has the effect of reducing stress and therefore should contribute to a diminution of flares.

Swimming is the only activity in which you might want to limit your participation, and that would only be because of the disapproval of other swimmers. If you enjoy swimming, many pools have designated times for people with special needs if you prefer, or are sensitive to the inquiring glances of others. If you do swim, you should shower as soon as possible to remove chlorine and other pool chemicals from your skin and apply a moisturizer right afterwards.

Relationships

Psoriasis may affect all relationships, particularly if the skin condition is very visible. Others may object to the messiness of the treatments, emollients and tar products, including the odor of some of the products. Stained clothing and skin flakes may be a problem for others to deal with. This requires a great deal of communication to foster an understanding of the condition and the treatments.

It is helpful if other family members go with the patient to the physician so that they may gain an understanding of the condition and the treatments.

Psoriasis may have an inhibiting effect on sexual relationships. While the condition does not affect the ability to have sexual intercourse, it may be considered an unsightly condition by some sexual partners. Also, they might be fearful that the condition is some kind of sexually transmitted disease. It is helpful to inform any sexual partner about the condition prior to becoming intimate; what it is, that it is not contagious, and what the treatments are, so that the partner will not be surprised by the condition of the skin. With adequate communication many people report no lack of acceptance in sexual relationships.

Depression

It is very easy to understand why depression would very easily be a companion to a skin condition. No one likes to feel that others find their appearance a cause for concern, and the fact that there is, at present, no known cure for psoriasis, certainly makes it readily understandable that it could add to someone's lack of self-esteem. It is easy to slip into a depression. It is well documented that a depressed individual will have a depressed immune status. Several studies have suggested that those who are depressed will take longer to recover from any physical illness. Depression also interferes with the mobilization of energy and can result in unwillingness to cooperate with treatments that may be tedious or that require physical effort. Taking an active, involved role has been linked with faster recovery from a variety of conditions, including cancer.

If the condition of your skin is causing you to feel a lack of joy, a feeling of dejection and a sense of constant unhappiness, it makes sense to get treatment for these emotions. It is wise to seek help from a professional who can help to expand your insight into ways of dealing with the skin condition and its effect on your emotions. Depressed people often see themselves as helpless or trapped in a hopeless situation and empathy, support, and compassion are often needed to help find the way out. A short course of psychotherapy or the help that can be found in a support group should be beneficial.

School and work

While it is unusual for psoriasis to begin at an early age, it can happen. Guttate psoriasis is the most commonly occurring type in school-age children.

The main difficulty for children with psoriasis is coping with the reactions of other children. It is not difficult to understand that children can be quite cruel to others when they see something they do not understand, particularly if the psoriasis is on a part of the body that cannot be covered.

If the child has psoriasis, it is best to make an appointment with the teacher and explain the condition and ask for the school's cooperation in helping the child gain acceptance, and informing classmates of the condition and what it means, particularly that it is not contagious.

Young children need assistance with treatments and it is important that sufficient time be made in the child's daily routine to care for the skin. It is important that the parent show patience, understanding and acceptance, so the child does not get the message that he/she and the condition are objectionable to the ones who should care the most, the parents.

Employment

Not many jobs are affected by having psoriasis but sometimes employers are. It is unlawful to discriminate against someone because of a skin condition unless it can be shown that the disease will affect the ability to perform the job.

There are some jobs where the condition could be considered a liability, especially if it is in an area that cannot be covered. Food service-type work, where the customers might be wary of being served by someone with a skin condition, and other occupations dealing with the public, such as receptionists and cashiers, are the kinds of jobs where employers might hesitate to employ someone with an obvious skin condition. Employment in situations where the skin is always wet, such as lifeguards or hairdressers, are occupations that possibly should not be considered for someone who has the condition.

Most employers need to be educated about the condition. It is the responsibility of the individual with psoriasis to be sure that the employer and co-workers are informed that the condition is not contagious, what causes it and how it affects the individual with the condition, before there is any problem so that unpleasant experiences can be avoided.

Menstruation/menopause

Menstruation and/or menopause do not appear to make any difference in psoriasis. Both are natural occurrences in the life of a woman and are regulated by changing hormonal levels. Psoriasis is not in any way related to these hormones.

Pregnancy

Pregnancy does not usually affect psoriasis. The condition does not affect fertility or the ability to bear children.

While psoriasis is inherited, it often skips generations. It is believed that the genetic blueprint is very complex, so it should not preclude anyone from considering parenthood for fear of passing on the condition to children.

9

What has helped others with psoriasis?

Because psoriasis is a condition for which there is no cure at present, and which has flares and remissions, there is a lot of folklore about what helps alleviate the condition. People who use some treatment and then have a remission are convinced that what they have done was helpful to them. Psoriasis has been around for centuries and there is a large body of ritual and folklore which has grown up around it. Most of the remedies are harmless, and if you would like to try them, go ahead. Perhaps something will be effective in alleviating the itching, pain or inflammation for you.

Many of the treatments that have been effective for others have not been proven effective by scientific study--nor have they been disproved either. There is no financial gain to be found in studying non-pharmaceutical treatments, therefore researchers have not studied things such as diet or simple herbs.

Homeopathy

Homeopathy is a medical specialty based on the principle that "like cures like," or the Law of Similars, which was put forth by Dr. Samuel Hahnemann, a nineteenth century German physician who is the father of the present day art of homeopathy.

When conventional medicine administers a vaccine, that is the logic of homeopathy at work. This method is ancient. In China, doctors would take scabs from the sores of smallpox victims and rub them on small cuts in the arms of those who were yet uninfected to, in effect, vaccinate them against the disease. This process gave them such a small dose of the disease that their body's immune system would go into high gear, making antibodies, and ultimately protecting them against any further exposure to the highly deadly disease.

Following this thinking, the homeopathic physician, using herbs, treats disease by exposing the person to something that will produce more of the same.

Homeopathic physicians usually treat psoriasis with herbs that in extreme amounts would be toxic. In the belief that an improperly functioning liver may be the basis of the skin condition, these physicians administer doses of a variety of herbs in a very controlled situation. Herbs such as comfrey and coltsfoot, which are known to be harmful to the liver in large doses (comfrey is known to impair liver circulation and coltsfoot has been shown to be poisonous to the liver--causing cancer in laboratory animals), are given to stimulate the liver to improve itself in response to the mild reaction caused by these herbs.

"In general, herbs produce only mild side reactions," says V. E. Tyler, PhD, a professor of pharmacognosy, at Purdue University School of Pharmacy. "Too much of *any* herb can be harmful," he says, "It is a good idea to see your physician before you self-treat with herbs."

Aromatherapy

More than 300 essential oils (distilled from herbs, fruits, flowers, roots, seeds, leaves, grasses, and other plant life) have been found to have antibiotic, antiseptic, antiviral, antifungal and anti-inflammatory effects.

Aromatherapists believe that smell controls our behavior in a number of ways. Using the sense of smell to gain access to the brain and the central nervous system, fragrances spark immediate reactions within the body. The therapist believes the odors released by these oils are nature's way of boosting the immune system; that they regenerate and stimulate cells throughout the body.

Proponents of aromatherapy feel that inhaling these essential oils can decrease anxiety, relieve tension and calm and sedate the user. They improve circulation to the skin and flush out toxins. Using this concept, herbs can decrease stress reactions in the psoriasis sufferer and thereby decrease the potential for flares.

Anxiety and tension:

2 drops marjoram, 2 drops sandlewood, 2 drops angelica and 1 drop jasmine. Sprinkle onto a tissue and inhale.

Other oils that are thought to counter anxiety include cedarwood, clary sage, geranium, juniper berry, lavender, lemon, rosemary, and ylang-ylang.

Skin care:

2 drops sandalwood, 1 drop lavender, 1 drop neroli and 1 drop Roman chamomile. Sprinkle onto a tissue and inhale. Or, add 2 teaspoons honey and spread the blend evenly over the lesions. After approximately 10 minutes, rinse off and apply an emollient.

Dr. George Zofchak's herbs

Dr. Zofchak, chiropractor, herbalist and naturopath, has spent a lifetime studying herbal remedies. His son now operates the business he began many years ago and sells hundreds of different herbs to customers all over the United States from his Tatra Herb Company in Morrisville, Pennsylvania.

Dr. Zofchak recommends the external application of a strong comfrey root decoction with goldenseal. "A strong tea is brewed and then cooled. Then a piece of soft clean white cloth is soaked in the tea and laid on the lesion. The liquid and the vapor of the herbs soak through the cloth to the skin. At the same time, take some capsules of the herb echinacea, which is an immunostimulant." Dr. Zofchak also recommends a tea known as Naturopathic, which can be purchased from the Tatra Herb Company.

For more information contact:

Tatra Herb Company
222 Grove St.
Morrisville, PA 19067
(215)-295-5476

Anyone interested in reading more about herbs and their use might read *Herbs that Heal*, by Michael Weiner, PhD.

Dr. John Douglass's elimination diet

In an attempt to find if dietary changes would make any difference in her psoriasis, Dr. Douglass's wife removed fruit from her diet (particularly citrus), and later, nuts, corn and milk. She found that this made a difference in her psoriasis, reduced the severity of the flare and lessened the frequency.

After seeing that this diet had been effective for his own wife, Dr. Douglass placed several of his patients on a similar program. The result was that quite a number of them improved. After further refinement, focusing on the acidic components of diet, he asked them to avoid all acidic foods such as coffee, tomatoes, sodas and pineapples--with good results.

Gluten-free diet

French physicians, studying the effects of diet on celiac disease, placed these patients on a gluten-free diet. Celiac disease is an inherited condition with an inborn error of metabolism. Individuals with this condition have an intolerance to wheat and rye proteins, which causes changes in the small intestine. These researchers report that people who had severe psoriasis in conjunction with celiac disease got a side benefit--their psoriasis was vastly improved. The theory is that gluten kicks off an abnormal response in the immune system, causing damage to the epithelial tissues. A gluten-free diet removes the protein found in grain such as oats, barley, rye and wheat.

Masada Dead Sea Mineral Bath Salts

Masada Dead Sea Mineral Bath Salts of Hollywood, California, claims to be able to provide these bath salts for use in your own bathtub. Their literature recommends bathing three to four times a week for 30 minutes in a tub to which four pounds of their product has been added. After the soaking bath, wrapping up in a warm blanket for 30 to 60 minutes is recommended.

Their literature cites the study of Dr. J. Arndt from West Germany who studied fifty patients treated with the salts in controlled administration for four weeks. Dr. Arndt claims healing was total in twenty-seven of the patients and there was marked improvement in twenty-two of the patients.

Masada Dead Sea Mineral Bath Salts can be obtained at:

P. O. Box 4767
North Hollywood, CA 91617
(818)-503-4611
Fax: (818)-503-3910

Soap Lake

Just as travelers go to the Dead Sea in Israel for four or five weeks to bathe in the water as a cure for their psoriasis, Soap Lake in Central Washington is a popular resort for those with psoriasis and arthritis. The water of Soap Lake has an unusually high mineral content and is located in a dry desert climate. Lake water is piped into many of the town's motels, and hot mineral baths are available. For more information, contact the local Chamber of Commerce:

Soap Lake Chamber of Commerce
P. O. Box 433
Soap Lake, WA 98851
(509)-246-1821

Omega-3 fish oil

British researchers found that fish oil, the equivalent of 5.5 oz. of mackerel per day (which provided Omega-3 fish oil) was beneficial. Dr. S. S. Bleehen, a dermatologist who co-authored a study which was reported in the *British Journal of Dermatology*, gave half a group of patients 10 Omega-3 fish oil capsules every day for twelve weeks while another half got capsules filled with ordinary olive oil. The result: there was almost no change in the olive oil users but there was a significant decrease in itching, redness and scaling in patients receiving the fish oil capsules.

Dr. Bleehen suggests that fish oil works by helping the body to more effectively process a substance known as arachidonic acid.

Dr. Vincent Ziboh, a biochemist and a professor of dermatology at the University of California, found, in a similar study, that sixty percent of patients had reduced itching, scaling and redness when they used Omega-3 fish oil.

Dr. Mindell's fish oil

Dr. Earl Mindell, professor of nutrition at Los Angeles' Pacific Western University and author of the book *Food as Medicine* also suggests that fish oil supplements may be an excellent treatment for psoriasis. "It really works," says Dr. Mindell. "About sixty percent of the people we studied responded well." He states that just eating more fish, especially salmon or mackerel, will do the same job.

Some groups of people appear to have a very low rate of psoriasis: Eskimos and Laplanders. These groups of people may, because of their isolation, have had little opportunity to enter into relationships with people who carry the psoriasis genetic potential, but also, they eat a diet high in fish and fish oils. These diets are high in the specific fatty acids recommended by Dr. Mindell and other researchers.

Dr. Robert Connolly's treatment

Dr. Robert Connolly, a chiropractor in Pontiac, Illinois, believes that sufferers of psoriasis need to take action to restore normal function of their liver and reduce toxicity in the body. He states that the liver is the great detoxification or cleansing organ of the body. He firmly believes that an improperly functioning liver is the common denominator in psoriasis. Dr. Connolly says, "When the liver does not function properly and does not detoxify waste products, the body will not function properly and this is responsible for the production of psoriasis."

He recommends self-massage twice daily of an area between the 5th and 6th rib at a point just underneath the nipple on the right side of the body which will stimulate the liver, plus accupressure in a circular motion on the inside of the knees twice daily, an area which is a liver-referral point, to cleanse and stimulate the liver.

Dr. Connolly says that one food sensitivity he has found in ALL his patients is pork. He recommends that it be excluded completely. He outlines a detoxifying diet that is free of pork (this includes all lunch meats, hot dogs, sausage and ham), limited in sugars, starchy foods, most flour and corn products and breakfast cereals. His cleansing diet is also restricted in certain vegetables and fruits and he recommends the use of a herbal formula known as D-Tox until improvement is noticed.

For a more detailed description of Dr. Connolly's regimen, how to massage the liver properly and details of the maintenance diet, write to him at:

Rt #1
Pontiac, IL 61764

D-Tox can be ordered from:

Vita Herbs
11911 Borman Drive
St. Louis, MO 63146
(800) 325-1108

Dr. James Balch's treatment

Dr. Balch, a urologist who writes a newspaper column and appears frequently on television, states in his book, *Prescription for Nutritional Healing,* that he believes outbreaks can be triggered by nervous tension and stress, illness, surgery, cuts, poison ivy, viral and bacterial infections, sunburns and several drugs.

He recommends that the diet be supplemented with Evening Primrose Oil, vitamin A emulsion, proteolytic enzymes, vitamin B complex, B12 and folic acid, thiamin and pantothenic acid with pyridoxine, vitamins C, D and E plus kelp, zinc, lipotropic factors, lecithin and a multivitamin and mineral complex containing magnesium and calcium chelate.

He suggests that lavender be used in a steam bath and poultices of chaparral, dandelion and yellow dock be applied to the lesions.

Dr. Balch recommends some dietary changes such avoiding fat, sugar, white flour, citrus fruits, red meat and dairy products.

He suggests that the diet should be fifty percent raw, uncooked. It is Dr. Balch's feeling that the less food is heated, and simply eaten in its natural state, the more nutrients will remain. He also strongly suggests that the diet for the treatment for psoriasis should include oils from sesame seeds and flaxseed, as both are rich in linolenic and linoleic acids, known to be beneficial to healthy skin.

Heat therapy

Researchers at Stanford University in Palo Alto, California, using ultrasound, raised the temperature of the patient's skin to 110°F for 30 minutes three times weekly. Dr. Elaine Orenberg reported that nearly all of the lesions treated with heat improved and most healed completely. It should be noted that it is possible to elevate and control skin temperature with moist warm compresses, taking care to avoid burning the area being treated.

Dr. Weirsum's treatment

Dr. Jeffrey Wiersum of Syracuse, New York is a nutritional physician who has treated patients with daily supplements of 25,000 IU of vitamin A, 800 IU of vitamin E and 50 mg of zinc. Dr. Wiersum's patients also applied vitamins A and E topically to their skin lesions. Dr. Wiersum says you should see results in six weeks.

Sunlight--available at no cost

Most people with psoriasis are aware that sunlight seems to help cure their lesions. The difficulty is that many people seem to think that if a little helps, then more will be more beneficial. Too much sun will make psoriasis worse, not better. Do not get sunburned.

Limit sun exposure to 15 minutes on each side of the body daily to begin and gradually increase the exposure by 15 minutes every second or third day to a maximum of no more than two hours. In southern parts of the US, exposure should be avoided between 10 AM and 2 PM, when the sun is the strongest. Time your exposure so that you will not fall asleep and awake with a severe sunburn and a worsened psoriasic condition.

It may take as long as four weeks before the sunlight improves the condition, so don't give up after only a few days. Protect your unaffected skin with sunscreen, or keep the unaffected areas well covered.

Band-Aid therapy--extreme occlusion

Dr. Ronald Shore of Johns Hopkins University noticed accidentally that skin that had been covered by a Band-Aid was free of psoriasis plaques. He confirmed this result by testing several airtight tapes and dressings on a number of psoriasis sufferers and found that the treatment was more successful than standard corticosteroid creams. Although Dr. Shore did not determine the reason for the success of this treatment, he states that he believes that the division of psoriatic cells are altered by a lack of air.

Science Digest reports that the application of adhesive tape has eliminated some lesions for a month or longer. They suggest that the success of this treatment is because excessive skin-cell replacement is controlled by hydration, sealing moisture in.

Vitamin E

There is a great deal of anecdotal evidence that suggests that vitamin E applied in liquid or ointment form and taken orally does help some people. Lecithin taken orally has been helpful. Oral niacin or niacinamide has been found beneficial. A dietary elimination trial has also been helpful, particularly when gluten foods have been removed from the diet (no wheat, rye, barley or oats).

Will acupuncture help?

Acupuncture was first used thousands of years ago in China. Its current popularity is possibly due to increased information about it and the arrival in the West of doctors trained in the technique.

Acupuncture involves the insertion of fine, sterile needles into the skin at appropriate acupuncture sites. Chinese teaching says that the insertion of the needles leads to chemical changes which stimulate certain nerves throughout the body. Western doctors who are trained in the technique use it mostly to treat acute and chronic pain.

One of the considerations that should be taken into account in the use of acupuncture is that when the needles enter the skin, it could result in a flare at that site, known as the Koebner phenomenon.

In individuals who have been helped by acupuncture, without a resulting Koebner phenomenon, it is speculated that it is because the needles are so fine they do not stimulate the skin to respond.

Acupuncture has been used to treat psoriasis with varying results and there has not been much interest in research into this treatment.

Well-known folk remedies

There are hundreds, probably thousands, of folk remedies for this skin condition. Since the first sufferer, people have tried many things to rid themselves of the flaky skin and itching. Here are some folk remedies that many people have claimed helped them. They are all probably harmless, some you might enjoy--and some might just possibly give you relief.

Try cod liver oil capsules, one a day for several months before relief is seen.

Take cod liver oil and linseed oil (flaxseed oil) capsules, two capsules of each just before bedtime.

Rotate Blue Star Ointment, cortisone-10 cream and Vitamin E cream. One every day to affected areas for three days and then start over.

Mineral oil applied liberally will restore the protective barrier of the skin.

Dissolve 1/2 cup of sea salt in 1 gallon of water. Soak the patches in the sea salt water several times a day. This is probably based on the knowledge that Israel's Dead Sea seems to work wonders for psoriasis sufferers.

In fact, the Dead Sea area of Israel has become famous as a healing resort. Patients spend weeks bathing in mineral-rich water and then soaking up the ultraviolet light from the sun. The Dead Sea is also said to be covered by a permanent haze that filters out the short burning rays of the UV spectrum while allowing the longer UV rays to pass through. Thus, a person can spend many hours in the sunlight without damage to their skin.

A study of almost 2,000 patients treated at the Dead Sea found that close to half of them had recurrences within four weeks after cessation of treatments.

Pat garlic oil on the affected area in the evening before retiring. Garlic is esteemed as a medicinal plant in many cultures, and recent research has documented some of the healing properties attributed to it in folk medicine. Garlic is a rich source of sulfur-containing compounds with biological activity.

Garlic is known to lower blood pressure, lowering cholesterol and blood fats while increasing the protective (HD) portion of cholesterol. Garlic is a powerful antiseptic and antibiotic, counteracting the growth of many kinds of bacteria and fungi that cause disease in humans. Furthermore, it enhances activity of the immune system, increasing numbers of natural killer cells.

You can get all these benefits simply by adding garlic to your food in any form. You can also buy a variety of garlic supplements, capsules of deodorized oil, or tablets.

Apply bloodroot to the affected area daily to speed healing.

Make a poultice of burdock root by boiling the leaves until most of the liquid has boiled off and then applying the hot, wet mass to the affected area until the leaves have cooled.

A number of folk remedies involve elaborate rituals which require preparing and appling one solution on odd numbered days and differing ointments on even numbered days. Often the preparation of the solutions and ointments require heating and straining and cooking a number of exotic ingredients. It is thought that these have some effect because they require the individual to pay scrupulous attention to the concocting and preparation of a long list of ingredients, and then make a careful examination of the condition of the skin at the time of a flare. The application of home-made preparations can be emotionally satisfying, whether or not they actually have any medicinal benefit.

Time spent in pursuing any creative hobby, such as creating a cream, cooking in the kitchen, growing herbs in the garden and then soothing yourself by applying your own creation in long hypnotic stroking motions can be stress-relieving. Whatever the reason, often these homemade preparations seem to improve the condition of the skin. So if someone gives you a recipe, accept the creative challenge; it might be interesting to try it and see if you get any results. You might be pleasantly surprised.

Prevention magazine asked individuals with a history of psoriasis to describe the treatments that have proven effective for them. Some of the replies included: drinking cherry or cranberry juice, following a butter-free diet, applying vitamin E skin cream, taking cod-liver oil, and the topical application of a concoction of aloe vera juice and L-lysine.

Individuals with severe eczema responded favorably when coffee and alcohol were removed from the diet. Since there appears to be a relationship between eczema and psoriasis, there is a possibility that removal of these two products entirely may help. Beer, nuts, chocolate or cocoa have also been known to aggravate skin conditions, so you might want to try eliminating them from your diet.

Soaking for 10 to 15 minutes in a tub of warm water to which half a cupful of baking soda has been added can relieve severe itching as reported in *The Lancet*, a prestigious British medical journal. Baking soda is a lot less messy than some of the other remedies.

Maintain adequate humidity in the house. During winter months in some climates it may be helpful to have a humidifier added to the heating system.

Nausea caused by the PUVA treatment can be aided by adding 1 teaspoonful of powdered ginger to boiling water and drinking this ginger tea after treatment. Ginger is a familiar culinary spice that has long enjoyed a reputation as a medicinal plant. Doctors in both China and India regard it as a superior medicine.

The tonic effects of ginger on the digestive system are clear: it improves the digestion of proteins, is an effective treatment for nausea and motion sickness, and strengthens the mucosal lining of the upper GI tract.

Other well-studied actions of ginger affect the production and deployment of a group of biological response moderators called eicosanoids, which increase healing and immunity.

Beta-blocker drugs are a frequently prescribed medication for high blood pressure and heart disease. In addition to helping control these conditions, beta-blockers produce quite a few side effects. One of the most troublesome is a skin reaction typical of psoriasis. *The British Medical Journal* reports that those who have had psoriasis previously, even only mildly, are certain to have a dramatic flare-up after starting on a beta-blocker. Fortunately, psoriasis brought on by a beta-blocker normally disappears soon after the drug is discontinued, and other medicine can usually be found to replace it. Beta-blockers are not the only medicines that induce psoriasis or cause it to flare up, and similar reactions can occur with the non-steroidal anti-inflammatory drugs (NSAIDs) that are widely used for arthritis and all sorts of aches and pains, including menstrual cramps.

Evening Primrose Oil is another oil that is derived from a plant source. The oil is quite different from the oils found in fish, the Omega-3 oils. It contains the essential fatty acids--gamma linolenic acid and linoleic acid--which are thought to be important in the production of natural oils which form the inner lining of the epidermal cells. Studies have shown that this type of oil is helpful for those individuals with eczema, not psoriasis. Some individuals who find that they do not have an adequate amount of these natural oils in their diet may benefit from supplementation with Evening Primrose Oil, but there are no scientific studies documenting that it is an aid in clearing psoriasis.

Quackery

Because there is as yet no definitive cause (although a hereditary failure of the immune system of the skin is the strongest candidate at present) and no absolute cure (at present, all treatments only suppress the symptoms), in a condition that has both remissions and flares, it is a prime area for quackery. Willingness to trade on the hope of sufferers has been, unfortunately, an opportunity that con men find irresistible.

An example is the claim of Vittorio Tosti that his multivitamin and mineral product could cure psoriasis. Despite testimonial letters and medical references which claimed to support the use of vitamins in psoriasis, his Vita-Skin Limited International--which marketed his product nationwide and in Canada and Italy--was denied permission to sell his product as a non-prescription drug since the FDA found his claims to be fraudulent.

There is no known cure, and advertisements by individuals who claim that they can cure the condition should be examined carefully, particularly if they are asking you to spend hard earned dollars on their cure or treatment.

If you find a treatment that seems particularly appealing, request back-up literature and check with your dermatologist and other experts before you involve yourself in any expensive and untried treatments.

10

Are psoriasis flares all about stress?

Stress can result from many things: a high-pressure occupation, relationships, financial difficulties, loneliness, crowds, traffic: the list can go on and on. Because of the complexity of the world, stress is experienced by everyone at one time or another.

Long-term stress often occurs when the situation that causes anxiety is not relieved. Even the wealthy, whom we all think should have no problems at all, experience stress. No one, no matter how content they seem, is exempt from stress. Some people even create their own stress: there may be nothing wrong, but they will find something to worry about.

Although everyone experiences stress, not everyone handles it constructively. The body can handle some stress, whether it is physical or mental. It must be coped with, and most people have the ability to cope. If the stress is short-term, then the chances are good that it will be dealt with. It is long-term stress that causes the body to break down.

Researchers at the University of Texas believe that when the brain is under stress, it produces an excess of the hormone ACTH. This hormone then inhibits the manufacture of white blood cells so vital to fighting disease.

A growing number of doctors believe that some common skin conditions, such as psoriasis, can be worsened or triggered by anxiety. While we are all aware there currently is no cure for psoriasis, longer and longer remission periods are something every patient can control rather than just long for.

With burgeoning new research into the role of a genetic defect in the immune system in psoriasis, more and more doctors are examining the role of stress in the triggering of psoriasis flares.

Recognizing early signs of stress and then doing something about it can make an important difference in the quality of life for the psoriasis sufferer.

Every year, one in three people in the United States experiences some form of skin disorder, and for a significant portion of these patients, emotional stress contributes to or worsens the episode, according to John Koo, MD, dermatologist-psychiatrist at the University of California, San Francisco. Dr. Koo estimates that 62 percent of individuals with psoriasis have an emotional trigger.

"More dermatologists are recognizing that the skin is an organ of emotional expression," says Bernard Kirshbaum, MD, clinical professor of medicine and chief of dermatology at Medical College of Pennsylvania. "Often, the skin is trying to express some unresolved internal psychic tension."

Researchers are just beginning to discover how and where emotions fit into the picture. Why is skin so responsive to emotions? "Skin is one of the body's primary organs of immunity," says Elizabeth Knobler, MD, assistant professor of clinical dermatology at Columbia University in New York. Negative, stressful or unresolved emotions may alter immune response, lowering resistance and allowing surface expression.

Chemical changes brought on by tension and anxiety may provoke not only psoriasis but acne, rosacea and vitiligo. Studies at Harvard University demonstrated that negative emotions stimulate the adrenal glands to overproduce the male hormones responsible for acne and rosacea. At Stanford University, researchers are looking at the stress-induced release of a specific substance in the body as a triggering factor for psoriasis.

Negative emotions can also increase nervous fidgeting, which may worsen certain skin conditions. Patients with patches of itchy, red, flaking skin are more likely than others to respond by itching and scratching in a stressful situation. Anxiety can enhance the perception of itchiness or pain, which lowers the itch threshold and triggers the scratch response, notes Dr. Koo. Scratching and rubbing the skin can release chemicals that cause further swelling in the upper layers of skin, exacerbating the condition.

Dr. Andrew Weil, MD, believes that because the skin has so many nerve endings it is a very frequent site for stress-related problems. He feels that conventional treatments for many skin diseases, especially topical steroid preparations, only suppress the condition.

He suggests lifestyle changes, particularly protection from the effect of sun damage, use of moisturizers immediately after a bath, elimination of cosmetic products containing dyes and other harsh chemicals, dietary modification to eliminate foods that may promote allergic and inflammatory changes, and an increase of the nutrients needed for healthy skin, hair and nails. He suggests supplementing the diet with antioxidant vitamins and minerals and with GLA (gamma-linolenic acid), an essential fatty acid of particular benefit to the skin. Most of all, he recommends that mind/body interventions should be tried to take advantage of the high level of innervation (supply of nerves) to the skin. Dr. Weil says, "I usually send patients to skilled hypnotherapists and guided imagery therapists. **All illnesses should be assumed to be stress-related until proved otherwise.** Even if stress is not the primary cause, it is frequently an aggravating factor. To say that a bodily complaint is stress-related does not in any way mean that it is unreal or unimportant; it simply means that time spent at stress reduction and relaxation training may be very worthwhile in terms of obtaining relief. Regardless of what other interventions you use, I recommend working with the relaxing breath, using mind/body approaches, and all relaxation methods that appeal to you in order to give the healing system the best possible chance to solve the problem that appears on the physical level."

If you suspect that you may be one of the individuals with psoriasis who has an emotional trigger linked to flares, the first step is to keep a diary of your daily ups and downs, activities and skin status. Do you find deadline pressures related to a flare? A family fight? A raise? The weather? Record good, bad and seemingly trivial events. At the end of a few weeks, you may begin to notice a pattern to your stress and skin upsets. Don't be surprised if there is a lapse of several weeks between the emotional event and the reaction that is evident in your skin condition. In his study of over 4,000 patients, dermatologist Robert Griesemer, MD, of Harvard University, noted lapses of anywhere from a few seconds (for hives and eczema) to up to two weeks (for psoriasis) between the likely trigger and an outbreak. Record keeping is the only way for you to gain insight into what kind of upset, pressure or irritation might trigger your skin problems.

While your skin condition may have a significant emotional component, you should take steps to treat the skin condition first. Psychological treatments should supplement, not supplant, medical care.

One of the biggest benefits from understanding your emotional triggers and then working to reduce their impact is knowing that you can do something about your emotional response to these triggers and this can aid in making you feel more in control of your disease.

Help yourself. Keep in mind that science is becoming more aware of the mind-skin link and actions to relieve pressure can help you keep your skin from being the outlet for your emotions.

Use physical activity

When you are nervous, upset or angry, one of the best known ways to release that pressure is through exercise or physical activity. Running, walking, or playing a sport, working at your hobby, or doing something that you enjoy are some of the activities that will be beneficial. There are a variety of activities that almost anyone can do: easy walking, Hatha yoga or tai chi (the slow muscle strengthening exercise of the Chinese) are excellent examples of exercise which will result in releasing muscle tension. Physical exercise can relieve that feeling of being up-tight.

Plan to make exercise part of your weekly routine. Any aerobic exercise, three times a week for at least twenty minutes each session can increase your ability to deal with stress and reduce muscle tension and anxiety.

A healthy body tolerates all kinds of stress much better than an unhealthy one. This is even more true for those with a skin condition that may be triggered by stress of all types. Regular exercise oxygenates the blood and the brain, increases alertness and concentration.

Exercise is a natural way to elevate endorphins, opiate-like compounds which are the body's natural pain killers. Natural pain-killers are a good way to interfere with the itch response and decrease the need to scratch the lesions. The runner's high is the well-known phenomenon that results from elevating endorphins through exercise.

If you begin an exercise program, begin slowly, particularly if you have not been exercising. If you have been sedentary, it is wise to check with your doctor before beginning an exercise program.

Practice abdominal breathing

Breathing is a very powerful way to energize and relax. When stressed, we breathe faster and shallower, making ourselves feel worse. To counter this reaction when you are anxious or upset, breathe deeply and slowly.

Many of us spend a lifetime breathing from the upper part of our chest, never fully aerating our lungs. We all need to counter this type breathing, which only increases tension rather than relieving it. Place a hand on your abdomen to make sure you are breathing in deeply (the abdomen expands as you breathe in). Then inhale to a slow count of four. Hold that breath for a count of sixteen--the optimum time to fully oxygenate blood and active the lymphatic system. Then exhale for a count of eight, while imagining the elimination of toxins and the circulation of oxygenated blood to your skin.

You may discover that this is difficult to do, particularly if you have been breathing only in the upper part of your diaphragm for a large portion of your life. You haven't experienced this abdominal breathing, so you don't know what it feels like. You must practice until it becomes comfortable. You may have to practice regularly to work up to holding your breath for 16 seconds. When you can, complete 10 breaths in this manner. You will notice a difference in how you feel. Try this kind of breathing in the morning while you are washing your face, on the way to a difficult meeting, or after an emotional encounter during the day.

When you feel fatigued, try this deep-breathing technique. While holding your breath, tap on your chest with your fingertips, moving your hand around so that the whole chest is covered. Try tapping your upper back also. Practice these methods regularly to invigorate your daily routine. Tapping stimulates circulation and body awareness. Try to feel the air in the areas you are tapping. Try it; it will make you realize how constricted your breathing is. This light tapping is both invigorating and relaxing. But remember, light tapping only.

When you have learned this relaxed breathing technique, it will help you in other stress-reduction techniques; whether it is hypnosis or guided imagery, you will find it benefits both experiences.

Share your emotions

It often helps to talk to someone about your concerns and worries. Talking to a friend, a family member, a teacher or counselor can help you see your problems in a different light. If you feel the problem is serious, you can seek professional help from a psychologist, psychiatrist or social worker.

Knowing when to ask for help may keep you from having serious emotional problems later.

Try Hatha yoga

Yoga is an ancient method of relaxation, breathing, meditation and mind-over-body control. There are whole books written on the subject, particularly the practice of Hatha yoga, the yoga of controlling the breath.

Yoga is a system of controlled breathing which has been practiced for centuries, and its structured stretching with slow deep breathing might be something you want to explore to increase your control over your own body and the way you breathe in times of stress.

Try meditation

Meditation, which was once thought to be of interest just to mystics and yogis, has entered the mainstream. Doctors, psychiatrists, and dentists are recommending that patients with anxiety learn to meditate.

There are numerous meditation techniques: Zen, Buddhist and transcendental meditation, (TM is probably the most popular with people in the western world). It doesn't matter what kind of meditation you do, they are all useful. The point is to be within yourself and let go of muscle tension and anxiety-provoking thought patterns.

The goal is to clear your mind and enjoy what you are doing while you are doing it, not to get to the end. The idea is to train both your mind and body if you want to have self-control and remain calm under pressure. Meditation has traditionally been connected to religious practices but that is not necessary for the benefits you might seek in your pursuit of relaxation.

In a study reported in the *American Journal of Psychiatry* it was found that 20 of 22 men and women who suffered from anxiety and anxiety-related conditions significantly reduced anxiety and depression after undergoing an 8-week meditation course. In this formal meditation practice, the patients were encouraged to develop moment-to-moment awareness, which led to a mindful calmness that undermined anxious feelings and gave them more of a sense of control.

Meditation is not a magic bullet, however. "It isn't recommended for crisis situations," says Kenneth Klein, a clinical psychologist who practices and teaches TM. "If your boyfriend or girlfriend breaks up with you, you are not going to feel like sitting down and meditating. But if you are too anxious to study or too stressed out to work, I'd recommend that you try it. TM helps you reintegrate so you bring more of yourself to the solution."

Klein suggests that anyone having problems with a superior at work, for example, take a break and meditate instead of drinking coffee. "It takes the edge off, and afterward you'll feel less angry and more able to deal with the situation. The point is not to get rid of the angry feelings but to use them productively."

Try biofeedback

Conventionally trained health care practitioners, including psychiatrists, nurses and physical therapists, have used biofeedback techniques since the 1960s to control autonomic nervous system functions that were traditionally viewed as unchangeable. Biofeedback uses sophisticated electronic machines with monitors and leads to give you a more precise picture of what is going on inside of you. You can learn to improve your health and wellness by watching a record of your heartbeat, pulse and blood volume track across the screen. Biofeedback has been used to treat many stress symptoms, including tension headaches, migraines, hypertension, insomnia, spastic colon, muscle spasm or pain, epilepsy, asthma and anxiety. It is very useful to understand that many of the reactions that we think of as automatic can be controlled through learned monitoring. It is possible to lower heart rates, decrease anxiety and anxious reactions, all by observing them, learning to control them and decreasing how they affect us--things we once thought were beyond our control. An example that can be easily understood is the mood ring, which changes color with the temperature of the hand of the wearer. A heat sensitive stone is the jewel in this type of ring, usually found in novelty stores. When the ring has a dark color, the wearer is supposedly in a dark mood. However, muscle tension throughout the arms control the temperature of the hands by restricting or increasing blood flow to the extremities. Using a mood ring, the wearer can learn to relax the arms, increase blood flow and find that the ring has changed to a lighter color, which supposedly indicates a happier mood. You can learn to relax arm muscle tension by becoming aware of it through this easy visualization tool. This toy can be an aid in understanding the theory behind biofeedback.

Buy an inexpensive mood ring, experiment with it; you'll learn to relax the muscles in your arms and in the process have a better understanding of your own tension.

If you are interested in biofeedback, your doctor can assist you in finding a professional trainer in your area.

Learn self-hypnosis techniques

Relaxation skills are just like any other skills. They require practice. You can purchase a relaxation/self-hypnosis tape from any book store or you can purchase specially designed audio tapes to relieve muscle tension and stress. These tapes will guide you through a series of progressive relaxation techniques and guided imagery.

It is possible to write your own relaxation script, record it and follow it, listening to your own voice instructing you on how to relax. You can add instructions to your self about your skin, seeing it healed and free of lesions. For best results, you should listen to your tape twice daily, morning and evening.

Enhance your relaxation experience by picturing your body relaxing. Use a color, symbol or sound--whatever is soothing to you.

You can use self-hypnosis to picture yourself taking a trip to a relaxing and safe place. A place where you feel comfortable and rested. Smell the scent of that place, hear its sounds, see its sights, feel the sensations and taste the tastes of it. Totally immerse yourself in that relaxing spot for a few minutes, give yourself skin-healing messages, then come back to the here and now, refreshed and relaxed.

Through hypnosis it is possible to control body temperature and heart rate. It is not some esoteric trick that can only be done by ancient mystics in some far-off land on top of a mountain. The mind is completely capable of expanding and contracting blood vessels, as can be proved with the inexpensive mood ring experiment, and with it comes the ability to raise and lower the heart rate. Picturing a pleasant day ahead and visualizing yourself as confident and relaxed can transport you through the day, manifesting a positive attitude in everything you do.

If you feel you need the assistance of a professional, your doctor can direct you to a professional medical hypnotist who can aid you in preparing yourself for self-hypnosis and guide you in performing this type of relaxation correctly.

Know your limits

If a problem is beyond your control and cannot be changed at the moment, work on accepting the situation for the present time, until such a time as you are able to make the change that is needed. Learn to say no to demands that overtax you.

Learn to manage time

Everyone has only twenty-four hours in each day. Some individuals manage to handle the day's tasks easily, some become stressed when they think they cannot accomplish all that they would like to. Time management skills are an essential foundation to managing stress, because they allow time to practice all the other techniques. Three basic time management skills are:

* priority setting
* elimination of low priority tasks
* decision making

Learn to say no. It is possible that this may require you to enroll in a course of assertiveness training and most local community colleges provide such courses. There are often such programs listed at your local library.

Build time into your schedule for interruptions and unforeseen occurrences.

Set aside time during the day for structured relaxation or listening to relaxation tapes. A relaxed person is more productive.

Take care of yourself

Get enough rest and sleep. If you are irritable and tense from lack of sleep or if you are not eating correctly, you have less ability to deal with stressful situations.

Nutrition

If you eat a lot of processed foods, frozen dinners, fast-food restaurant meals, or follow low-calorie diets, you may be shortchanging your body and your brain. You probably don't realize it, but continually drinking coffee or soft drinks or missing meals weakens your body's natural resistance to anxiety. During periods of stress it is particularly important to bolster your diet by eating balanced meals every day and possibly adding a vitamin supplement.

A well-balanced diet builds stress resistance in a number of ways. It increases physical endurance, increases resistance to disease and promotes increased emotional stability.

Roger Williams, in *Nutrition Against Disease,* describes an adequate diet as follows:

Amino Acids: Amino acids are the building blocks of protein. They are essential for a number of reasons: they build body tissues; they supply food fuel for the body whenever insufficient fats and carbohydrates are consumed; they help maintain normal blood sugar; they assist in the transport of various minerals and vitamins; and they assist in the acid-base balance of the body. Protein is needed for the health and formation of muscles, hormones, membranes, glands, enzymes, skin, plasma, teeth, antibodies, ligaments, hair, fingernails, bones, cartilage, hemoglobin, brain and nerve cells.

Vitamins: Vitamins are essential to life. They contribute to good health by regulating metabolism and assisting the biochemical processes that release energy from digested food. They are considered micronutrients because the body needs them in relatively small amounts compared with other nutrients such as carbohydrates, proteins, fats and water.

Enzymes are essential chemicals that are the foundation of human bodily functions. They are activators in the chemical reactions that are continually taking place within the body. Vitamins work with these enzymes as coenzymes, thereby allowing all the activities that occur within the body to happen quickly and accurately.

Of the major vitamins, some are water soluble and some are oil-soluble.

Vitamins B and C

Vitamin B is actually a complex of several vitamins, including B1, B2, B3, B6 and B12, PABA, as well as folic acid, choline and inositol. These are water soluble vitamins, which means they are not stored in the body and therefore must be supplied in sufficient amounts at all times--especially when the body is under stress.

Even though the B vitamins should be supplied in the diet in quantities sufficient to support normal health, this supply can be inadequate under stress. Stress is anything that causes extra tension--emotional or physical--such as drugs, alcohol, chemicals, excessive fatigue, noise, infections, disease and anxiety.

The B vitamins are found in whole grain cereals and breads, dark green leafy vegetables, beans and soy beans, brewer's yeast, wheat germ, poultry, beef and liver.

Vitamin C, another water soluble vitamin, is essential to the body for the formation of collagen in the body; collagen is a protein substance that cements the cells of the body together to make tissue. It is important and necessary for the development of healthy capillaries, bones, cartilage, teeth and connective tissue; to protect the body from infection; to aid the adrenals in the production of cortisone; to assist in the absorption of iron from the intestines.

This vitamin is an antioxidant: it helps to neutralize foreign substances, chemicals and poisons in the body. The body's need for vitamin C increases greatly during times of stress; again, this is stress in any form--emotional or physical--such as during an infection.

Without vitamin C we would have scurvy, a disease that was common in sailors on sailing vessels who were at sea for lengthy periods at a time and had no access to fresh fruit. Scurvy is seldom seen now in the western world. However, minor forms of this disease can be seen in bleeding gums, the tendency to bruise easily and the tendency to sinus infections, allergies and hayfever.

Vitamin C is present in citrus fruits and dark green leafy vegetables.

Vitamins A, D and E

These three vitamins are fat soluble, that is, fat is necessary in the diet for these vitamins to be properly absorbed by the body.

Vitamin A is an antioxidant which contributes to sight, resistance to infections, and the maintenance of healthy skin, bones and mucous membranes.

Vitamin D is called the sunshine vitamin because exposure to the rays of the sun produce this vitamin which is then stored in the liver. It is needed for the body to properly utilize calcium and phosphorus which are both important for strong bones and teeth.

Vitamin E is an antioxidant and it plays a role in the protection of vitamin A, as well as body fats.

Vitamin A is widely distributed in yellow vegetables and fruits such as carrots, cantaloupe, sweet potatoes, apricots, dark green leafy vegetables, eggs, milk, fish liver oils and liver.

Vitamin D can be found in fish liver oils, eggs and fortified milk.

Vitamin E is available from vegetables, oils, grains, eggs, liver and meat.

Minerals: Like vitamins, minerals function as coenzymes, enabling the body to quickly and accurately perform its activities. They are needed for the proper composition of body fluids, the formation of blood and bone, and the maintenance of healthy nerve function.

Minerals are naturally occurring elements found in the earth. Rock formations are made up of mineral salts. As rock and stone are broken down into tiny fragments by millions of years of erosion, dust and sand accumulate, forming the basis of the soil. Besides these tiny crystals of mineral salts, the soil is teeming with microbes that utilize them. The minerals are then passed from soil to plants, which are then eaten by herbivorous animals. Man, in turn, obtains these minerals for use by the body by consuming these plants or herbivorous animals.

Minerals belong to two groups: macro (large) and micro (trace or small) minerals. Bulk minerals include calcium, magnesium, sodium, potassium, and phosphorus. These are needed in larger amounts than trace minerals. Although only minute quantities of trace minerals are needed, they are just as important for good health. Trace minerals include zinc, iron, copper, manganese, chromium, selenium and iodine. Because minerals are stored primarily in the body's bone and muscle tissue, it is possible to overdose on minerals if an extremely large dose is taken for a prolonged period of time.

Vitamins cannot function without the assistance of minerals. Minerals work together as a group rather than individually. They work in conjunction with hormones, enzymes, proteins, carbohydrates, fats and vitamins. They are required for the proper overall mental and physical function of the body and they help to build and maintain the entire structure.

Calcium

Calcium is the most abundant mineral in the body: about 99 percent of the calcium in the body is found in the bones and teeth, the other one percent is in the soft tissues and the blood--this lowly one percent has a great impact on the nerves.

Calcium is found in milk, dairy products, green vegetables, cereal and bread.

Magnesium

Magnesium is a natural tranquilizer for the nervous system. It is required for protein and carbohydrate metabolism. Signs of magnesium deficiency are similar to those of a hangover: sensitivity to noise, tremors, twitching, rapid heartbeat, aching muscles, fatigue, depression, and irritability. It is the only electrolyte which has a higher level in the brain fluid than in the blood plasma.

Magnesium is available from whole grain breads and cereals, green leafy vegetables and milk.

Potassium

Potassium is vital for the proper functioning of nerves, heart and muscles. It is important for chemical reactions within the cells, and aids in maintaining stable blood pressure and in transmitting electrochemical impulses. In addition, it works with sodium to maintain the body's water-salt balance.

Potassium is available from dairy foods, fish, fruit, poultry, vegetables and whole grains.

Phosphorus

Phosphorus is important in nearly all physiological chemical reactions within the body. It is necessary for normal bone and tooth structure and for the transmission of nerve impulses, and is necessary for the metabolism of fats and carbohydrates.

Phosphorus deficiency is rare because it is found in most foods. Significant amounts of phosphorus are in asparagus, corn, dairy products, eggs, fish, dried fruit and sunflower seeds.

Iron

Iron is found in the red blood cells as part of the hemoglobin, and hemoglobin is the protein that carries oxygen to the body tissues.

Iron's sources include whole grain cereals and breads, wheat germ, dark green leafy vegetables and beans.

Zinc

Zinc is required for protein synthesis and collagen formation. It promotes a healthy immune system and the healing of wounds.

Zinc is found in legumes, poultry, seafood, whole grains, brewer's yeast, egg yolks, lima beans, sunflower seeds and mushrooms.

The remaining minerals have a number of complex enzymatic functions in the monitoring and repair of body systems, and are found in either a multi-mineral tablet or in a varied diet.

Because there are other obscure nutrients such as phenols, flavones and lutein which science does not as yet fully understand, it is necessary to eat a diet rich in a variety of fruits and vegetables.

Chronic stress, whether environmental, physical or emotional, often results in a need for the anti-stress vitamins, B and C. These two vitamins are rapidly utilized any time the body is stressed and need to be replaced with regular nutritious meals.

Unfortunately, for many of us, the first thing to suffer during periods of excessive stress is most often the diet. Stress and anxiety tend to interfere with the digestive system, which decreases its activity during these times, leaving us with an upset stomach. In addition, those foods which have a low nutritional content but often have a high emotional value, such as chocolate or sugary treats, are quite often used as a coping device. When the diet goes by the wayside during anxiety, the body is less able to resist the effects of stress and that results in increased anxiety.

The body and the brain can be likened to a machine: without proper fuel it does not run well or efficiently. It is not necessary to count calories and grams of fat and carbohydrates to be well nourished. There are hundreds of books on nutrition and well-balanced meals in any book store or library.

However, those with psoriasis lesions, which opens the body to an easy route for infection, should avoid fad diets or those diets which are likely to put additional stress on the nervous system. Most people, even without any skin problems, will feel better on a nutritionally balanced diet.

When you are experiencing a period of high stress, pay strict attention to your diet. In addition, if you know that you are facing a stressful period, pay extra attention to seeing that your body and brain are well nourished.

Food cravings are well known to have a mood connection. Women typically crave sugar-fat combinations. Eating sugars and starches increase the presence in the brain of serotonin, the brain chemical that is the body's own natural antidepressant.

Fat cravings may be a need to stimulate endorphins, those opiate-like compounds that are the body's natural pain killers and are triggered by eating fats. When endorphin levels are low you will feel anxious, depressed and your appetite for fat (as well as sugar) is activated. These dietary antistress foods give a temporary endorphin lift plus a serotonin lift. But beware, there is a backlash effect: If you raise blood levels of sugar and fat excessively, they will only fall drastically in a few hours, leaving you feeling more anxious and depressed.

Weller and Walker, authors of *Orthomolecular Nutrition* state that: "Every tissue in the body is affected by nutrition. Under conditions of poor nutrition, the kidney stops filtering, the stomach stops digesting, the adrenals stop secreting and other organs, including the skin, follow suit. Somehow, many doctors labor under the false belief that somehow brain function is completely separate from the body and its nutrition. Nothing could be more wrong. The mind-body connection is very important. An undernourished body cannot provide a well-nourished brain, and without a well-nourished brain stress will soon affect the body. This is a cyclical effect and when the body is affected, it will appear in that most essential organ, the skin."

Sleep

Chronic sleeplessness can increase anxiety symptoms and interfere with health, relationships and the ability to function effectively. Because chronic sleep problems can be due to a medication or a medical condition, it is best to discuss sleep problems with your physician. Difficulty in sleeping is quite often due to poor bedtime habits or thinking patterns which interfere with the ability to get to sleep.

If your sleep is poor or interrupted, or you waken early feeling fatigued, it is possible that the problem may be depression and should be discussed with your doctor.

Sleeping medications are habit forming, are only for short-term sleeplessness, and should only be taken after attempts have been made to improve your bedtime habits. Prescription sleeping medications can alter normal sleeping patterns and suppress REM sleep. The body becomes tolerant to some forms of these drugs, and higher and higher doses become necessary, leading to dependency. Quite often, the use of prescription sleeping pills for a short-term period of sleeplessness can lead to long-term sleep problems.

Application of your nighttime psoriasis emollients should be done routinely. If you do not allow enough time before going to bed you will find yourself rushing to get the task completed and you may find that you have stimulated your skin rather than soothed it. An easy, relaxed application of the emollient should decrease the itch stimulation rather than arouse it. Treat your skin gently, kindly, lovingly so that it can respond in kind.

Melatonin is lowered in the morning by light, and darkness increases the levels of this brain chemical which regulates our sleep cycles. Maintain a healthy internal biological clock by going to bed and arising at the same time each day and do not sleep in on the weekends or days off. Naps are all right if they are taken early enough in the day, are not for more than thirty minutes and do not appear to be the cause of sleeplessness.

If you are a shift worker and must make schedule changes, do so gradually. One week before the change, go to bed an hour earlier each night in a darkened room. At the beginning of the week you may have a little trouble going right to sleep but by the end of the week you should be waking at the right time for your shift.

Avoid stimulants for three to five hours before bedtime. Caffeine and heavy meals are not beneficial to good sleep. Avoid alcohol. While many think of alcohol as a night cap, a relaxing drug, even moderate amounts of alcohol can disrupt sleep and often cause a backlash of sleeplessness in the early morning hours.

Reserve your bed for sleep and sex. If you read, watch exciting television, eat, work crossword puzzles in bed, you are setting up a subconscious concept that your bed is for all kinds of other activities.

Make the bedroom inviting to sleep in. Make the window treatments heavy enough to keep out light and noise. It is easier to fall asleep in a room that is dark, quiet and well ventilated.

Establish a bedtime routine by setting up a conditioned response. If you regularly wash your face, brush your teeth, set out your clothing for the next day, wind the clock, walk the dog, apply your emollients in calm, rhythmic strokes--do all things in a regular routine order. This will become your conditioned response that triggers your body to go to sleep after these things are finished. Whatever activities you choose for your conditioned response, such as a bath, praying or meditating, remember to choose only relaxing activities. Avoid anxiety-arousing activities such as paying bills, watching horror movies or listening to loud, energizing music.

If you go to bed and find that you cannot fall asleep, do not stay in bed worrying about the fact that you cannot get to sleep. After no more than twenty minutes, get up, do something that you regularly find relaxing in some other part of the house. Read or watch television or some other quiet activity until you begin to feel sleepy; only then should you go back to bed.

Exercise just before attempting to sleep will interfere with sleep. Even three to five hours before bedtime, heavy exercise will interfere with your ability to sleep. However, light exercise, such as a walk around the block after dinner, will improve the amount of good sleep in the early part of the night.

Lying in bed worrying about tomorrow's problems will definitely keep you awake, even if you are physically exhausted. Get up, go to another room and make a creative plan to deal with that something you are worrying about. If this is a future event, role play the various things you think could or might happen, and decide how you will handle them. Visualize yourself handling the difficulty well. Once you have done this, go back to bed and practice one of your relaxation techniques. If you find yourself drifting back to thinking about the problem, repeat your creative plan to yourself and resume your relaxation exercise.

If you find that you routinely do this type of worrying once you go to bed to sleep, then establish a time before going to bed to formulate a creative plan. Once you are in bed with a plan well thought out, use relaxation techniques to assist you to sleep.

If you find that you awaken in the middle of the night worrying about something and can't get back to sleep, get up, go to another room and do something calming before attempting to sleep again.

If you are going through a period of sleeplessness, take the time just before going to bed to engage in a brief relaxing activity, such as reading, listening to calming music and perhaps having a cup of warm milk or herbal tea. It is helpful to have things prepared ahead of time. Have one of the tapes or CDs you would like to listen to already on the stereo. Have something out to heat the milk in should you think you are going to want it. Have something available to read that is calming, such as a book of poetry. This should take no more than ten minutes, in which time you will allow the physical symptoms to quiet themselves. Then go to bed, relax with pleasant pictures in your mind and go to sleep.

11

Approaches to the management of itching and pain

Itching and occasional pain is a common complaint of those with psoriasis. Both pain and itching are unpleasant sensory or emotional experiences associated with actual or potential tissue damage. They are highly subjective experiences influenced by personality traits and emotional factors, and can be acute or chronic.

Constant itching can cause substantial anxiety, which can cause physical tension and increase the feeling of itchiness. Psychological approaches to the management of both itching and pain attempt to disrupt the experience by alleviating anxiety, either directly via relaxation techniques or indirectly by restoring a sense of control. These approaches also help ease the depression and sense of helplessness which can accompany the physical discomfort.

Perceived control plays an important role in mental health in general, and in reducing itch and/or pain in specific. The finding that pain and/or itching is substantially reduced when one feels a sense of control is a well-documented fact.

Specific psychological approaches to itch/pain management include relaxation, distraction, hypnosis, guided imagery and biofeedback.

Relaxation

Originally used to manage anxiety, it is important in pain and itch management as well. Anxiety and discomfort go hand in hand; by reducing anxiety, both can be diminished. Relaxation also directly affects the physical process by reducing muscle tension and diverting blood flow. A component of relaxation is controlled breathing. Focusing attention on the breath serves not only as a form of distraction, but leads to a general slowing down of metabolism with an attendant over-all sense of tranquillity.

Distraction

Essentially, this causes both pain and itching to recede into the background of awareness by directing the focus toward an attention-getting stimulus. The stimulus is unique to the individual's interest at any particular time. A broad range of mental and physical activities can be selected as options from which the individual can choose. Many find that focusing on something that they are very interested in, such as a sport or a game, can take the mind off of the itchiness of the skin. Distraction, however, is usually of short duration and is sensitive to personality factors. Distraction is more effective when used in conjunction with other techniques.

Hypnosis

Hypnosis is one of the oldest and most effective psychological interventions available. It employs a combination of techniques, all of which have beneficial effects. The rationale given is that all hypnosis is essentially self-hypnosis, and it instills a sense of control which can be effective. First of all, the individual must be willing to be hypnotized. Hypnotic induction begins by engendering a state of relaxation. This, in itself, relieves anxiety and physical tension. Hypnosis further diverts the mind from the pain or the itch and thus serves as a distraction. An additional factor unique to hypnosis is the altered state of consciousness that is induced. In this state, suggestibility is increased. Expectations for pain/itch relief are more likely to be met. After a series of hypnotic training experiences, the individual is given the tools and can proceed to use them on his or her own to control the pain/itch experience.

Try guided imagery

Dr. Andrew Weil, in his book *Spontaneous Healing,* says he believes that no disease process is beyond the reach of guided imagery and visualization therapy. He states that it is best to work with a trained professional, at least initially, to ensure you are using these therapies correctly. Guided imagery and visualization can enhance the effectiveness of other treatments, including drugs and surgery.

Guided imagery provides a sense of control, engenders a state of relaxation and diverts attention from pain and itching. With an instructor, the individual is instructed to visualize a peaceful, relatively unchanging scene and is encouraged to use the senses of sound, sight, touch, smell and taste to make the image as vivid as possible. In this very safe environment the individual works on visualizing the psoriasis healing, not returning, fading in redness and with lesions growing smaller and smaller until they disappear entirely. Guided imagery is best suited to those with vivid imaginations. Those with problems imaging may do better using biofeedback.

"I feel so trapped, I feel like I'm in a cage."

"The itching is driving me crazy, I tell myself I am going to keep my hands off my head but I seem to be unable to control them."

These are some of the comments made by patients in a guided imagery class, based on the images they picture when they think about their psoriasis. When these mental images are vivid enough that a picture can be formed in the mind, guided imagery may be a treatment of choice for that individual.

Someone who is capable of having these images of their skin condition can also do the opposite: visualize the plaques becoming quieter, decreasing in size and eventually disappearing.

When our eyes are open, we are drawn to scenes that we perceive outside of ourselves. When our eyes are closed and there is silence, images and thoughts come to us about our inner state. Dreams, daydreams, and fantasies are examples of how our mind pictures what we think and feel. Guided imagery can have three basic valuable uses:

Becoming more receptive: To help become more aware of feelings, dissatisfactions, tensions, and images that are affecting body functioning.

Healing: To help erase bacteria or viruses, build new cells to replace damaged ones, make rough areas smooth, hot itchy areas cool, sore areas comfortable, tense areas relaxed, bring blood to areas that need nutrients or cleansing, make moist areas dry or dry areas moist, bring energy to fatigued areas and enhance general wellness.

Problem solving: To consult with one's intuitive source of wisdom in a structured way or break down barriers to clear thinking.

Body relaxation facilitates the flow of internal images, so when guided imagery is used it is helpful to first assist the person to a relaxed state. A quiet comfortable place is mandatory. Reading a relaxation script or playing a tape of relaxing music or words is often helpful.

Images can be negative and disturbing, or relaxing and health-producing: the choice is yours. A properly trained guided-imagery practitioner can help people focus on developing positive, healing images.

The trainer asks the person to describe the itch or the pain. After the image is identified, they work together to produce a more positive, satisfying image. Together they might visualize the plaques floating away, and the person releasing whatever emotion is most troublesome and stepping forward to a new skin. Or she/he might be asked to remove the skin layer by layer until new clear skin is revealed. The person creates the image, the trainer only guides the process.

Guided imagery is a powerful tool that bypasses the brain where obsessive repetitive or negative thoughts can affect the body and the functioning of the mind. Once the person is taught to get in touch with body sensations, relaxation has already begun to occur.

Anyone interested in guided imagery might read *Seeing With the Mind's Eye* by Samuels or contact a local office of the American Psychological Association for a further referral to a trained practitioner.

Train yourself to stop worrying

It is a well known fact that it is not possible to think two thoughts simultaneously. When worries come into your mind, tell yourself "STOP!" The concept of thought stopping is based on the theory that we are all engaged in self-talk during our waking hours. If we can only have one thought at a time, it will change our thinking if we stop negative thoughts from starting. Notice when a disruptive thought comes into your mind and either picture a stop sign or mentally say to your self, "STOP." If there is nothing that you can do about it at the moment, it is a waste of time to recycle the worry over and over in your mind, only causing yourself more and more frustration. When you begin to think about your skin, particularly if the thoughts are negative, such as, "Everyone is looking at my elbows. They are probably wondering what is wrong with me" that STOP message can be effective in keeping this type of thinking from developing further. Once you are aware that you have given yourself a message to stop the negative thought, it needs to be followed with some positive thinking, such as, "I am better than I was yesterday, I am able to control my skin and make it better."

Develop coping skills

Coping skills are very similar to assertiveness training. They are statements which can be rehearsed prior to a tension-provoking situation and then can be used during an uncomfortable encounter. They work well as preparation in combination with structured relaxation.

For example.

Something has upset you. Instead of continuing to go into the situation, you begin by performing some relaxed abdominal breathing. Instead of running through a list of retorts you might have made or how you could have gotten even, you begin self-talk in a positive manner. This can be rehearsed before-hand for specific situations that you know always cause you stress, or generically for the types of stress that increase your anxiety.

Make time for fun

Schedule time for both work and recreation. Play can be just as important to your well-being as work. You need a break from your daily routine just to relax and have some fun.

Your skin won't be the only part of you that will be appreciative. Everything is better in our lives when we don't become workaholics, noses to the grindstone, hunched over our work day-in and day-out. A person who is enjoying life and has a variety of activities that are interesting will feel better, look better and enjoy better mental and physical health.

Participate in outside activities

Get involved in something and become a participant. Offer your services to some charitable organization. Help yourself by helping other people. Not only is being involved a great distraction from what is bothering you, but volunteer work can help you maintain perspective on what it is important in life.

It is OK to cry

A good cry can be a healthy way to bring relief to your anxiety. Take some deep breaths, they also relieve tension.

Find time to laugh

Laughter can make you feel much better. Its therapeutic value is well-known. Norman Cousins in his book *Anatomy of an Illness*, documented his recovery from cancer and how he self-medicated with hours of Marx Brothers' old movies and cartoons. Cousins believed he literally laughed his disease away.

Create a quiet place all your own

A quiet country scene painted mentally can take you out of the turmoil of a stressful situation.

Change the real scene, which may not be to your liking at the moment, by reading a good book or playing beautiful music to create a sense of peace and tranquillity.

Eliminate caffeine

People who drink too much coffee may experience palpitations, jitters and gastrointestinal distress. Anyone under stress should avoid caffeine. Caffeine is routinely used by scientists to induce panic attacks in clinical experiments. Caffeine is a stimulant sufficient to affect the way both the brain and body respond and function. Specifically, caffeine constricts the blood vessels, restricting oxygen and nutrient flow--particularly to the extremities and the skin.

Replace caffeine with a herbal tea. Just sitting down and having a cup of relaxing tea can aid you to relax and re-charge.

Eliminate nicotine

Nicotine, the stimulating ingredient in cigarettes, is absorbed through the mucous lining of the mouth and the lungs, where it is passed into the bloodstream and circulated to the brain. Nicotine triggers a variety of responses in the nervous system. It acts on the control center in the brain in a number of vital functions. It increases the output of the heart, constricts the blood vessels and elevates blood pressure. Just like caffeine, nicotine reduces the blood flow to the skin, reducing necessary nutrients that repair and heal, as well as the skin's germ fighting cells, which help in the prevention of infections and in the healing process of traumatized skin.

Eliminate alcohol

Alcohol has effects on all body systems and it can create feelings of anxiety and cause insomnia, rather than relaxing you. While it may seem to be relaxing at the moment of its use, its metabolism requires and finally uses up all the body's B vitamins, which are necessary for the proper operation of the nervous system. Alcohol makes the skin feel warmer, which makes itching worse. In addition it reduces inhibitions, allowing you to scratch freely, irritating and aggravating the already existing fragile skin condition.

Eliminate illegal drugs

Both cocaine and amphetamines are stimulants that interfere with the chemical functioning of the brain. Over time, these drugs replace the natural brain chemicals which normally regulate both mood and perception. After prolonged use, the brain may cease to produce the neurotransmitters that counter irritability and other elevated responses, resulting in excessive anxiety and its related mental states.

Marijuana intoxication can contribute to a feeling of unreality or depersonalization. This unreality can cause many people to experience a feeling of loss of control with a resultant anxiety.

Because someone with psoriasis needs to eliminate anxiety and have a feeling of being in control, the use of stimulants, such as cocaine and amphetamines, and the use of marijuana, which some may think of as a pain-killer, all contribute to increased anxiety and stress in the long-term, conditions which are not beneficial to those serious about gaining control of their skin.

12

Jennifer's story--learning to cope

"Finally, after long periods of resisting any help I started going to a specialist, a dermatologist. I learned a lot from him about the condition but I really didn't want information, I just wanted a cure. I wanted something simple, just a daily pill or something like that. I wanted to wake up in the morning and find that my skin had cleared up. That didn't happen. He changed me from treatment to treatment, looking for the best thing for me. Sometimes it seemed to help, sometimes it didn't. I would cooperate for a while and then I'd get sick of the baths and the smelly stuff and become very angry at everybody. I'm sure I was not a lot of fun to live with."

Again Jennifer went through great periods of depression when she refused to take care of her skin, refused to take any medication and just gave up on everything. "I just sat around in my room feeling sorry for myself. One of the first treatments I had was steroids and the results were very dramatic. The redness went down right away, the itching stopped and I got very excited," she said. "But when I stopped using it, the psoriasis came back, even worse than before. Living with any chronic disease is difficult; I'm sure that people with long-term pain or a terminal, disabling disease would think that just having something wrong with your skin--they would be willing to trade. But this condition is ugly and unpredictable and inspires a lot more stares, pointing and whispering than sympathy. The emotional effect can be devastating."

Jennifer smiled, "I felt like my life was over. I couldn't swim, I couldn't wear pretty clothes. I had lost my boyfriend and doubted that I would ever have another. I didn't even want to think about a job. Who would hire me?

"Every time I would come around and cooperate with the treatments my parents were very understanding and sympathetic. My mother helped me apply the stuff I had to put on my lesions and I changed the bedding and washed the sheets myself. Then, when it looked like I wasn't going to get better and I began to give up on my treatments, they got disgusted with me again. My father would yell at me to stop feeling sorry for myself. But I couldn't. I felt very sorry for myself.

"Finally, the dermatologist called to find out why I hadn't been back to keep my appointments and my mother talked to him about my depression. My doctor put me in touch with a support group and my parents literally dragged me to the first meeting.

"I didn't want to go in. I didn't want to sit in a room with a bunch of freaks, moaning about how terrible they looked and how much they itched and how bad the world treated them. But I went and sat with my arms folded across my chest, feeling very angry that I had been dragged there. I couldn't stop myself from hearing what they said, though. I went to about four or five meetings before I said anything myself, I just sat there and listened to them. But finally, I began to realize that these people understood what I was going through and as I looked around I could see that there were people there whose condition was worse to look at than mine.

"I began to relax. I began to realize that this was reality. I needed to get myself under control, to take action myself, to be responsible for the condition of my own skin. I guess I was finally growing up, accepting my condition and realizing that these people at this meeting were very much like me. Finally, I began to take control. To learn what worked for me and what didn't. But the most important thing I learned was that remissions and flares were my responsibility. When I took control of my reactions to stressful conditions and made sure that I got sufficient rest and ate properly, my psoriasis got better. I listened to the others, I learned from their years of experience."

Jennifer's psoriasis support group

This is what Mary, a young blond bank executive said: "I came hoping to find a magical cure. I have been coming to these meetings for about a year now and I still am waiting for that magic. But I'm adult enough to guess there probably isn't any and there isn't going to be any very soon. But coming here has helped me. I know that I'm not alone. I can talk about my experiences, can have a few laughs at what has happened to me and to others. Before I started to come to the group meetings I thought I was the only one with this condition. Now I know that others have problems in their lives because of psoriasis and sometimes it helps just to know that. I also learn things from others who have had the condition longer than I have. I've learned that despite what I've been through I'm never going to give up hope. Maybe there will be a cure soon. I don't know but I have to keep on looking, actively looking for a treatment that works for me. I search out possibilities and follow up on the folk remedies others tell me about. I ask questions, read books and articles, go to the library. I know that some doctors think I'm difficult, obnoxious, but that's OK, I keep on questioning."

Debbie, a middle-aged housewife, told the group: "I was visiting my husband's family for the first time.

We were staying in their spare bedroom and my psoriasis was very bad at the time. I felt just as if I was covered in scales from head to toe. Every time I moved I could feel skin flakes falling off of me and I just knew that all of my husband's relatives were staring at me. I would be the first up in the morning and the last to bed at night because I wanted to vacuum up my flakes, not leave a mess for other people. I wanted to be sure that there wasn't anything on the bedspread, it was a family heirloom. I had brought my own bedding, my own towels, and a little hand-held vacuum cleaner.

" Well, it turned out that my mother-in-law thought I was doing all this cleaning because I thought her housekeeping was sub-standard. She was absolutely furious and very offended and told my husband she didn't think much of his wife!

"We all laugh about it now. This was quite a learning experience for me. I realized that it is a lot better to explain to people right from the very beginning. You can avoid a lot of complications in relationships by doing that. A lot of years have passed and my husband's family have come to accept my skin condition, just like I accept my mother-in-law's weight and my father-in-law's snoring that shakes the whole house. I have made a lot of new friends among the people I have met at the meetings and they have helped me, by example, to live with the condition. I have met people at these meetings who have now been healed and that gives me hope."

Harold, a balding man who manages a small copy machine business, told the group: "I have had a number of experiences that have really strengthened my long-standing belief in mind/body interactions and I now pay a lot closer attention to my mental and emotional life than I ever did before I developed psoriasis.

"I was traveling in a sales job when my psoriasis developed and I really couldn't take proper care of myself on this drive. The psoriasis got really bad between my buttocks and I was miserable sitting in the car for hours at a time. In the evening I would slap on my lotion and fall into bed and try to sleep in a strange bed every night. As it got worse, I got more and more anxious about it. By the time I got home several weeks later, it was raging out of control and so was I."

Harry's wife Marilyn spoke up: " I was really into alternative therapies then, and I knew this nurse who was practicing guided imagery at the time. I begged Harry to go to see her, just listen to the ideas she had."

Harry laughed, "I called Deborah, more to appease my wife than for my own sake. Under Deborah's guidance I went to a place out in the desert I know and love (all in my mind, you understand). We spent quite a time getting me relaxed and comfortable with this so-called mind trip. It was an idea that I wasn't too comfortable with at the beginning but I worked on it. After I was settled, she asked me to pick one lesion that was bothering me the most. Well, you would have thought I would pick one on my face, because that was what I was showing to the public but I didn't, I picked the one between my buttocks, the one that was giving me so much discomfort.

"'Put your mind right there,' Deborah said, 'and tell me what you see.' I saw a mass of swirling angry energy, puffing up in big red balls of anger.

"'Listen to it and see if it has anything to say to you.' I thought all this was silly, especially thinking of my skin between the cheeks of my bottom talking to me--but I had agreed to try it. Immediately words popped into my mouth. 'It says it cannot leave my body by going into the atmosphere,' I responded. 'I want it to leave my body but it can't. It has to go inward and be absorbed.' I waited to see if Deborah would laugh at my remarks, but she didn't.

"'If that is what it needs to do, what should you be doing?' Deborah asked.

"Immediately I had the answer. 'Well, I suppose I should not be sitting in a car all day long, sweating. I should be lying in the sun in the backyard with my buttocks exposed and I should be resting more. But,' Harry protested, 'that's just common sense. I'm not taking care of my condition, and it is making me madder than hell!'"

Deborah suggested that they go back to the desert place that Harry could visualize in his mind and there he could take all his clothes off and lie in the sun, concentrating the sun's rays onto his lesion.

"I couldn't think how this could have helped me, but I went to bed relaxed and confident that night that my body was going to take care of itself. The next morning, I could see that my lesion on my buttocks was better; less inflamed, less angry-looking. In addition, I had made a decision to quit the sales job," laughed Harry.

"I'm not saying that this is some kind of a miracle cure but if interactive guided imagery can cure back pain, stomach ulcers and cure all other kinds of skin infections why shouldn't it be able to turn anything around? I suggest that everyone try some kind of mind/body technique because they are unlikely to cause any harm and might do themselves a lot of good. My wife says I'm a New Age person now, but that's OK. I'm a believer and I know that when I get stressed and start trying to do too much, my skin reminds me that it is time to slow down and take some time to make some lifestyle changes and now I do that by visualizing with guided imagery."

Beverly, the wife of a successful surgeon, went from dermatologist to dermatologist who each prescribed steroids for her psoriasis. She wanted to try some alternative forms of treatment but her husband, a surgeon schooled in traditional medicine, was strongly opposed.

"I would get better with the treatment but when I went off, my lesions came back, worse than before. After a while I became really depressed and I spent most of my time lying in bed or soaking in soothing baths."

Beverly's husband's profession left him little time for home life and she felt isolated and depressed. "Without telling my husband I went to a hypnotherapist. I knew my husband wouldn't like it because he would be afraid of the idea of anyone taking over my mind. I got a little hot plate and I put it next to my tub and I would make some herbal tea to sip, which I found very soothing.

"I was pleasantly surprised by my experience with the hypnotherapist. She taught me relaxation methods and I began to practice them regularly while

I lay in my tub and sipped my tea. After about six weeks I began to see some improvement. Then suddenly the improvement accelerated and has continued steadily. My hypnotherapist believes that conventional medicine had only offered me suppressive therapy. She feels that any disease of the skin should be assumed to have an emotional basis until proven otherwise, because these systems are the most frequent sites of expression of stress-induced imbalances. Mind/body interventions combined with lifestyle change can often allow the body to heal itself completely from these conditions."

Beverly laughed, "My husband doesn't believe any of this but now that I am better and feel like going out and doing things, he is making more time for me and our relationship has improved greatly."

When asked why she continues to come to the group she replied, "Because I believe so strongly in the mind/body connection, I want others to hear my story and maybe be helped. It is so little to ask that I do this, how can I not come?"

Louise, a young postal worker, says, "One of the first times I came to these meetings I heard someone say that they considered psoriasis a gift. I was stunned. I couldn't believe that anyone would say such a thing. But the more I thought about it, the more I could see that maybe she was right. I know that I'm not the same person I was before psoriasis came into my life. I've been on a search and I've made significant changes in my life: relationships, a job, diet, life-style habits. These changes have been necessary on the way to personal growth but change is always difficult. Psoriasis had forced me to look at issues and conflict in my life in the hope that they would disappear. This person told me about Dennis Potter, the author of *The Singing Detective* who has written so eloquently about his 27 year battle with psoriatic arthropathy. Potter writes that the disease made him confront questions others ignore and has forced him to redefine himself. I've come to realize that seeing this as a misfortune is an obstruction and seeing it as a gift has given me the opportunity for personal growth and development."

Lois spoke up: "They brought in some speakers, experts in controlling pain. I have a lot of pain with my psoriasis and that was very helpful to me. They talked to us about cognitive methods to relieve pain. I thought that was a big word, but when they began to explain the non-drug methods that work, I realized that it made sense. Research scientists from the City of Hope National Medical Center offered many options, which others here are already using, such as humor, guided imagery, auditory stimulation, progressive relaxation, meditation or prayer, and music.

"The speakers explained each of them like this:

"Humor makes pain more tolerable by placing it at the periphery of awareness. Laughter, naturally occurring and effortless, controls pain by reducing tension and increasing the production of endorphins.

"Guided imagery uses the five senses to create pleasant images as a substitute for the sensation of pain. A guided image therapist helps create the image with places and things that are familiar to the patient.

"Auditory stimulation involves listening to tapes with nature sounds. It works with the sense of hearing and gets the individual to concentrate on the natural environment, encouraging relaxation.

"Progressive relaxation is the active tightening and releasing of large muscle groups while noting the differences between the sensations of tension and relaxation. The goal is to increase the ability to identify even mild tension and reduce it.

"Meditation or prayer focuses attention and alters the level of awareness. It can be structured or unstructured, involving mentally directed feelings and thoughts in a relaxed state through silent conversation or chants, or focusing on an idea or object.

"Music therapy can help divert the person's attention and help to gain a sense of control.

"Some of these ideas were new to me, others were not, but they all made sense. I realized the choice of cognitive method is primarily based on trial and error and a lot depends on the personality and life experience of the individual. It really helped to have professional people tell me that they had clinical experience with these methods and they weren't just esoteric mystical stuff."

Jennifer says, "Coming to this group has been so helpful to me. I'm accepting myself now with the imperfections, limitations and defects that are mine, just as everyone else has their set of imperfections, limitations and defects. I've learned a lot of practical information here too, things that the dermatologist doesn't tell you because he doesn't have the time or doesn't have the experience himself of dealing with the condition in the real world. I'm trying guided imagery, hypnosis, and a couple of other things that seem to help others. I know now that there is great research going on concerning genetic engineering. I'm hopeful again and that has taken me out of depression and into life again. I'll be going away to college in the fall, I'll be sharing a room in a dorm with a complete stranger and I think I can handle it--and I'm looking forward to it."

Will there ever be a cure?

Recent research has led to a new understanding of the biochemistry of the skin, and as a result there are new treatments being developed which reduce the thickened skin, reduce itching and decrease inflammation.

There is a recent early pilot study at the Laboratory for Investigative Dermatology at Rockefeller University in New York which has the potential for discovering a cure for psoriasis.

Using work pioneered by Dr. John Murphy of University Hospital in Boston, scientists took the molecule that causes deadly diphtheria and modified it genetically. "Diphtheria has three main domains—one of which tends to bind to all cells in the body. We removed that part of the molecule and in its place inserted interleukin-2, a protein which attaches to activated immune cells," Dr. James Kreuger, a researcher at Rockefeller, told a reporter.

Dr. Kreuger and his fellow scientists thought that psoriasis was a disease caused by auto-immune malfunctions. They speculated that they could fight the disease by tricking the activated cells that cause the overproduction of skin cells into attacking the so-called fusion toxin. The activated cells would ingest the toxin part of the molecule and then die.

As a result of this work, researchers have reported that eight of 10 people with severe psoriasis had lessened symptoms in the preliminary test of this new drug which is expected to alleviate rather than cure the disease. This new drug may help at least some people with the chronic skin disease. It is the strongest evidence to date that misguided immune attacks underlie psoriasis. Seragen's drug will ultimately consist of an immune messenger molecule chemically linked to a potent toxin.

It has been often speculated that an immune disorder was the causative factor in this genetically inherited disease, but it has never been proven, according to the National Psoriasis Foundation.

In this pilot study, 10 patients with severe psoriasis were given the fusion toxin treatment in 15-minute intravenous infusions five days a week, and then were allowed to go home for 23 days. The patients returned for another 5-day treatment, and four of the 10 showed striking improvement; another four showed moderate improvement within four to eight weeks.

"This is a very important result in pointing toward the future direction for therapy," said James Krueger, the Rockefeller University researcher and senior author of a report in the journal *Nature Medicine*. In the study of this new product, Seragen, four of the 10 had striking reductions of scaliness, itching and other symptoms, with afflicted patches of their skin appearing to return to normal. Another four had moderate improvement. This new product appears to selectively knock out certain immune cells, and the patients with the most improvement were ones in which abnormal immune-cell activity in the skin was most reduced.

A spokesman for Seragen, the biotechnology company interested in development of the treatment, told a reporter, "People with severe psoriasis said they would be willing to undergo this type of delivery if they could be assured that it would end their psoriasis. However, we are looking into other delivery methods which are more readily provided, such as patches and inhalants." In its present form, the combination acts like a bomb addressed to activated T cells, the immune cells that may trigger psoriasis. The selective attack on the immune system isn't expected to cause serious side effects, with the main side effects in this limited study being flu-like symptoms, including headache, fever and chills. The manufacturer's spokesperson says he hopes that the drug potentially could alleviate psoriasis for a considerable length of time, perhaps many months.

Further studies are presently in the planning stages, but it would appear that this genetic engineering approach could be the breakthrough that many sufferers would like to see happen.

Glennis McNeal, spokesperson for the National Psoriasis Foundation, said, "We find this development very exciting. It is a whole different approach to the disease. There is always a need for new treatments because individuals with psoriasis tend to build up resistance to therapies."

Researchers James Elder and Gary Fisher are investigating the transforming growth factor in the skin of those with psoriasis. They have found that TGF messenger RNA and protein are much more abundant in lesional psoriatic skin than in normal-appearing skin of psoriatic patients, or in the skin of individuals without psoriasis. This discovery could lead to a further understanding of the growth of the epithelial cells and a way to interfere with the overgrowth.

Scientists P. Saiag, B. Coulomb and C. Lebreton, reporting in *Science*, developed a skin equivalent model to study the outgrowth of epidermal cells in psoriatic skin. They attempted to suppress the growth in cultures through the introduction of fibroblasts (a cell of connective tissue). They found that the primary defect(s) in the excessive growth lay within the very selective skin cells. They anticipate that this skin equivalent model may be useful for further studies of the disease.

Elof Eriksson, a plastic surgeon and researcher at the Brigham and Women's Hospital in Boston has developed research that takes advantage of a hormone called Epidermal Growth Factor (EGF), a wound-healing compound made by humans and other animals. Having isolated the EGF gene several years ago, scientists have been able to mass produce the hormone inside cultured, laboratory-reared cells, and use the substance as an experimental wound-healing drug. They gave the cells in a wound extra EGF genes so the cells could make large quantities on their own.

Eriksson and his colleagues took thousands of microscopic gold pellets a fraction the size of a human skin cell and coated each pellet with EGF genes. Then they used a special "gene shotgun" to blast the tiny DNA-coated beads directly and painlessly into fresh skin wounds in pigs, whose hide is almost identical to human skin.

Tests showed that the genes developed in the pigs' skin cells (EGF concentrations jumped almost 200-fold in the wound site), creating a healing treatment right where it was needed. Healing time was reduced by 20 percent.

A great deal of further testing is required before the treatment can be used on humans, but researchers believe that in the future the delivery of "cocktails" of wound-healing genes may be used in the treatment of skin ulcers, deep scarring wounds or skin diseases such as psoriasis.

Researchers James Tomfohrde, Alan Silverman and Robert Barnes have discovered that a gene involved in psoriasis susceptibility is localized to a particular human chromosome (the part of the cell that carries the genes). Their study demonstrates that, in some individuals, psoriasis susceptibility is due to a variation at a single major genetic locus. This research makes it possible to focus on a particular area of the genetic makeup of the psoriatic malfunction, and narrows the field for further study in the field of genetic engineering.

More research is needed to isolate the particular gene(s) involved in psoriasis, but once found, it will then be necessary to determine how and why it/they do not work properly and what specific abnormality is produced. If this particular abnormality can be located, it may be possible to design treatments to correct the way the gene(s) works, to remove it/them, defuse it/them, or replace it/them completely with a correct-performance gene, through genetic engineering. Orthodox and the unorthodox may be used together, with a combination of holistic and mainstream practice. This is all good news for the stress reduction concepts of treating psoriasis.

It may be that the future of science and medicine, together with genetic engineering, can hold out the possibility for the eradication of psoriasis!

Where can you find more help?

In a historic decision, the U. S. government has decided to take a closer look at alternative medicine by establishing the Office of Alternative Medicine. The office, part of the National Institutes of Health, is devoted solely to studying alternative treatments, such as acupuncture. "We will be testing things to see if they have scientific value," says the director, Dr. Joseph Jacobs.

Because many forms of unconventional care use positive thinking and other psychological factors, scientific studies might not yield results. This is a dilemma that Jacobs acknowledges, conceding that medicine may have to change the way it measures healing.

The American Academy of Dermatology
P. O. Box 4014
Schaumburg, IL 60168-4014

The Skin Research Foundation of California
(310) 828-8969

The National Psoriasis Foundation
6600 S.W. 92nd Avenue, Suite 300
Portland, OR 97223
(503) 244-7404

American Association of Biofeedback Clinicians
2424 Dempster Avenue
Des Plaines, IL 60016

Biofeedback Certification Institute of America and Association for applied Psychophysiology and Biofeedback
10200 West 44th Avenue, Suite 304
Wheatbridge, CO 80033

Academy for Guided Imagery
P. O. Box 2070
Mill Valley, CA 94942
(415) 389-9324

American Society of Clinical Hypnosis
2250 East Devon Avenue, Suite 336
Des Plaines, IL 60018
(708) 297-3317

There are psoriasis organizations worldwide, in dozens of countries. Most of them can be found by looking for the organization in a major city under the name of the country, followed by the word *Psoriasis*.

For example:

Israel Psoriasis Association
P. O. Box 13275
Tel-Aviv, Israel

Norsk Psoriasis Forbund
Grenseveien 86 A
0663 Oslo, Norway

What is the National Psoriasis Foundation?

This organization is a tax-exempt, nonprofit organization in the USA which works solely to aid people who have psoriasis, and is dedicated to educating people about psoriasis. In 1991, the NPF received the American Academy of Dermatology's *Excellence in Education Award.*

NPF provides extensive services to people who have psoriasis, their families, and to the public. It publishes two national newsletters, the *Bulletin* which keeps members current on treatments, details updates on research and provides fresh ideas on self-care; and *Pharmacy News* that highlights interesting articles on a variety of consumer-related issues, announces new or unique products and lists over-the-counter and prescription medications, all to help people stay informed about new and existing treatments, psoriasis research, and self-care. Educational booklets, video tapes and audio cassette tapes are available which address a number of psoriasis topics. NPF sponsors conferences and workshops to bring people face-to-face with medical experts, scientists and pharmaceutical representatives in an effort to help them gain control over their disease.

In addition, NPF supports and stimulates research by lobbying Congress for federal funding of skin research, and offers its own research grants to stimulate new ideas and attract more investigators to the field of research in psoriasis.

NPF initiated and continues to support the National Psoriasis Tissue Bank. This bank is a repository of genetic information on families with a history of psoriasis. This information is available to researchers worldwide to help them in the search for the gene(s) linked to psoriasis.

NPF also sponsors basic research meetings where scientists can exchange scientific information and identify new leads for research.

The organization will provide an array of educational booklets on specific psoriasis topics, and two of these booklets are also published in Spanish.

In addition, NPF contracts with a pharmacy to bring its members quality medications and products at the lowest possible prices.

The staff is available to aid those with difficulties in insurance claims, emotional or psychological difficulties, location of specific treatments, complications with employment or any issue that might be aided with counseling or further assistance.

You can find a local support and education network of individuals with psoriasis through NPF.

NPF maintains a listing of physicians in the United States recommended for treating psoriasis and psoriatic arthritis and the location of PUVA or UVB resources.

The Foundation knows the location of all psoriasis day care centers, treatment centers, and climatotherapy sites.

National Psoriasis Foundation
Tel: (503) 244-7404
Fax: (503) 245-0626

Index

C

D

E

N

O

P

Notes

Notes